Embedded Pharmacists in Primary Care

Embedded Pharmacists in Primary Care

Editors

George E. MacKinnon III
Nathan Lamberton

MDPI • Basel • Beijing • Wuhan • Barcelona • Belgrade • Manchester • Tokyo • Cluj • Tianjin

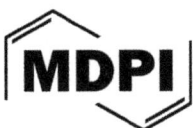

Editors
George E. MacKinnon III, PhD, MS, RPh
Medical College of Wisconsin
USA

Nathan Lamberton, PharmD, BCPS
Medical College of Wisconsin
USA

Editorial Office
MDPI
St. Alban-Anlage 66
4052 Basel, Switzerland

This is a reprint of articles from the Special Issue published online in the open access journal *Pharmacy* (ISSN 2226-4787) (available at: https://www.mdpi.com/journal/pharmacy/special_issues/Embedded_Pharmacists_Primary_Care).

For citation purposes, cite each article independently as indicated on the article page online and as indicated below:

LastName, A.A.; LastName, B.B.; LastName, C.C. Article Title. *Journal Name* **Year**, *Volume Number*, Page Range.

ISBN 978-3-0365-0170-3 (Hbk)
ISBN 978-3-0365-0171-0 (PDF)

Cover image courtesy of Wisconsin School of Pharmacy.

© 2021 by the authors. Articles in this book are Open Access and distributed under the Creative Commons Attribution (CC BY) license, which allows users to download, copy and build upon published articles, as long as the author and publisher are properly credited, which ensures maximum dissemination and a wider impact of our publications.

The book as a whole is distributed by MDPI under the terms and conditions of the Creative Commons license CC BY-NC-ND.

Contents

About the Editors . . . . **vii**

Preface to "Embedded Pharmacists in Primary Care" . . . . **ix**

George E. MacKinnon III
Concept for Embedded Primary Care Pharmacist Practitioners (PCPPs): A Disruptive Value-Proposition
Reprinted from: *Pharmacy* **2020**, *8*, 195, doi:10.3390/pharmacy8040195 . . . . **1**

Katherine J. Hartkopf, Kristina M. Heimerl, Kayla M. McGowan and Brian G. Arndt
Expansion and Evaluation of Pharmacist Services in Primary Care
Reprinted from: *Pharmacy* **2020**, *8*, 124, doi:10.3390/pharmacy8030124 . . . . **5**

Kyle Turner, Alan Abbinanti, Bradly Winter, Benjamin Berrett, Jeff Olson and Nicholas Cox
How a State Measures Up: Ambulatory Care Pharmacists' Perception of Practice Management Systems for Comprehensive Medication Management in Utah
Reprinted from: *Pharmacy* **2020**, *8*, 136, doi:10.3390/pharmacy8030136 . . . . **15**

Jarred Prudencio and Michelle Kim
Diabetes-Related Patient Outcomes through Comprehensive Medication Management Delivered by Clinical Pharmacists in a Rural Family Medicine Clinic
Reprinted from: *Pharmacy* **2020**, *8*, 115, doi:10.3390/pharmacy8030115 . . . . **23**

Renee Robinson, Cara Liday, Anushka Burde, Tracy Pettinger, Amy Paul, Elaine Nguyen, John Holmes, Megan Penner, Angela Jaglowicz, Nathan Spann, Julia Boyle, Michael Biddle, Brooke Buffat, Kevin Cleveland, Brecon Powell and Christopher Owens
Practice Transformation Driven through Academic Partnerships
Reprinted from: *Pharmacy* **2020**, *8*, 120, doi:10.3390/pharmacy8030120 . . . . **35**

Camlyn Masuda, Rachel Randall and Marina Ortiz
Pilot Study: Evaluating the Impact of Pharmacist Patient-Specific Medication Recommendations for Diabetes Mellitus Therapy to Family Medicine Residents
Reprinted from: *Pharmacy* **2020**, *8*, 158, doi:10.3390/pharmacy8030158 . . . . **49**

Jordan Spillane and Erika Smith
From Pilot to Scale, the 5 Year Growth of a Primary Care Pharmacist Model
Reprinted from: *Pharmacy* **2020**, *8*, 132, doi:10.3390/pharmacy8030132 . . . . **57**

Jennie B. Jarrett and Jody L. Lounsbery
Trends in Clinical Pharmacist Integration in Family Medicine Residency Programs in North America
Reprinted from: *Pharmacy* **2020**, *8*, 126, doi:10.3390/pharmacy8030126 . . . . **65**

Manmeet Khaira, Annalise Mathers, Nichelle Benny Gerard and Lisa Dolovich
The Evolving Role and Impact of Integrating Pharmacists into Primary Care Teams: Experience from Ontario, Canada
Reprinted from: *Pharmacy* **2020**, *8*, 234, doi:10.3390/pharmacy8040234 . . . . **73**

About the Editors

George E. MacKinnon III Ph.D., MS, RPh, FASHP, FNAP has engaged in clinical practice, research, teaching, and academic administration through joint academic appointments in medicine and pharmacy at several educational institutions during the past 30 years. Dr. MacKinnon has helped found and accredit four academic pharmacy programs, in three states. Dr. MacKinnon's previous appointments include vice president of academic affairs with the American Association of Colleges of Pharmacy in Alexandria, Virginia, and the director of global health economics and outcomes research of Abbott Laboratories. Dr. MacKinnon received a Bachelor of Science in Pharmacy and a Master of Science in Hospital Pharmacy, from the University of Wisconsin-Madison School of Pharmacy. He completed two years of post-graduate clinical pharmacy residency training at the University of Wisconsin Hospital and Clinics. Dr. MacKinnon earned a Doctor of Philosophy degree in Educational Leadership and Policy Studies from Loyola University, Chicago. He is a registered pharmacist in three states. As an educator, administrator, researcher, and clinician he has been intimately involved in developing programs in the areas of teaching, service, and research in the health professions. He continues to demonstrate the value of pharmacists in various models for primary care, comprehensive medication management, population health, pharmacogenomics, and pharmacoeconomics. He is the Editor of the textbook Understanding Health Outcomes and Pharmacoeconomics. He has been recognized as a Fellow of the American Society of Health-System Pharmacists (FASHP) and a Distinguished Scholar Fellow of the National Academies of Practice (FNAP).

Nathan Lamberton, PharmD, BCPS joined the Medical College of Wisconsin School of Pharmacy in 2017 as a Clinical Assistant Professor. Dr. Lamberton has a clinical practice site with Columbia St. Mary's Family Medicine Residency in their outpatient Family Medicine Center. He received his PharmD from the Albany College of Pharmacy and Health Sciences. Prior to joining MCW, Dr. Lamberton completed a combined PGY-1 Pharmacy Practice/PGY-2 Ambulatory Care (Family Medicine Focus) pharmacy residency and a longitudinal two-year Faculty Development Fellowship with UPMC St. Margaret in Pittsburgh, PA. Dr. Lamberton's primary interests include interprofessional education and chronic disease state management. He maintains active involvement with the Society of Teachers in Family Medicine (STFM) through the Pharmacist Faculty Special Project Team.

Preface to "Embedded Pharmacists in Primary Care"

The work environments and expectations for primary care physicians' daily activities include spending a significant amount on chronic care management, including managing complex medication regimens. Multiple resources have projected shortfalls in primary care providers in the United States. Ergo, a future should be envisioned where pharmacists are embedded in primary care settings, as primary care pharmacist practitioners (e.g., PCPPs). The benefits of such providers include enhanced medication adherence, fewer adverse drug-related events, reduced inappropriate healthcare utilization (e.g., emergency room visits, hospitalizations, office visits), improved clinical outcomes, total reduced cost of care (assessing pharmaceuticals as part of this), greater patient satisfaction, and higher CMS star ratings (thus impacting reimbursements).

Given the projected shortage of primary care providers (PCPs), the explosion of high-cost specialty pharmaceuticals, future use of pharmacogenomics in precision medicine, and value-based reimbursements, the addition of a pharmacist to most physician practices will be financially prudent, if not essential. Appropriately leveraging the role of the pharmacist in primary care settings to achieve better health outcomes in all patients and achieve not only the triple but quadruple aim is a value proposition worthy of exploration by all members of the healthcare team. This collection of works embody this spirit and desire to articulate and demonstrate the value of embedding pharmacists in primary care practice settings.

George E. MacKinnon III, Nathan Lamberton
Editors

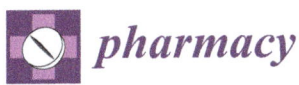

Editorial

Concept for Embedded Primary Care Pharmacist Practitioners (PCPPs): A Disruptive Value-Proposition

George E. MacKinnon III

School of Pharmacy, Department of Family & Community Medicine, Institute for Health Equity, Genomic Sciences and Precision Medicine Center, Medical College of Wisconsin, Milwaukee, WI 53226, USA; gmackinnon@mcw.edu

Received: 15 October 2020; Accepted: 17 October 2020; Published: 23 October 2020

The work environments and expectations for the daily activities of primary care physicians are daunting and often include spending a significant amount of time related to chronic care management with complex medication regimens, medication reconciliation, and the documentation within the electronic medical record (EMR) of these medication related issues. For a variety of reasons, there has been a reduction in physicians that are pursuing primary care roles in the United States. The Association of American Medical Colleges (AAMC) 2020 Report projected shortfalls in primary care ranging between 21,400 and 55,200 physicians by 2033 [1]. Supplanting of physicians by advance practice providers (i.e., nurse practitioners and physician assistants) will not meet the growing healthcare needs and required expertise to best serve the growing United States population. The time for the addition of an experienced healthcare provider to the primary healthcare team has come, and that provider is the pharmacist.

Given this projected shortage of physicians and the explosion of high cost specialty pharmaceuticals and growing use of biomarkers and the future of pharmacogenomics in precision medicine, the addition of a pharmacist to most physician practices will be clinically and financially prudent, if not essential in time. A future should be envisioned where pharmacists are embedded in primary care settings as primary care pharmacist practitioners (PCPPs).

As pointed out in the 2014 publication [2], physician burnout is associated with lower patient satisfaction, reduced health outcomes, and it may increase total healthcare costs. As such, dissatisfied physicians are more likely to prescribe inappropriate medications that can result in inexpensive complications [2], thus an opportunity for pharmacists to engage at the point of prescribing (e.g., in the primary care clinic setting) could provide a welcomed new member to the primary healthcare team.

Clearly, embedded pharmacists in primary and specialty care could assume other roles as called for in the 2011 U.S. Surgeon Report [3]. This call, which is now almost ten years since, has also been in part supported by the American Medical Association (AMA) as exemplified in that it has produced a tool to help physicians improve patient care called "STEPS", which includes a relevant module (*Embedding Pharmacists Into the Practice: Collaborate with Pharmacists to Improve Patient Outcomes*) [4].

Having pharmacists embedded in primary care is not revolutionary, rather, it is evolutionary. In the United States, there are multiple models of where pharmacists are practicing within the full scope of their licensure and are included as credentialed members of the primary healthcare team. The Veterans Administration (VA), Indian Health Service (IHS), and Department of Defense (DoD) have recognized the unique and valuable contributions that pharmacists can provide to beneficiaries for the past 40 years. The Middleton VA in Madison, Wisconsin was highlighted in *USA Today* where there is one clinical pharmacist per six physicians, accounting for over 25% of patient encounters with chronic medical conditions seen by an embedded pharmacist in primary care clinics [5]. As reported, there is a desire to increase the ratio to one pharmacist to three physicians in primary care at the Middleton VA.

On a commercial level, Kaiser Permanente has led this effort in the Western states for the past twenty years, and this has been occurring in other states within larger academic medical centers. Why this trend? Simply stated, chronic care management utilizes medications to treat patients, and who better to add to this team than the healthcare provider who has more education and knowledge about medications, the pharmacist?

To address these forthcoming challenges, our health profession academies, in particular medicine and pharmacy, must collectively think differently (or disruptively), but collaboratively. The described intentions are to create, in conjunction with our medical colleagues and other healthcare providers, disruptive practice models and teams of the future that leverage appropriately, so the role of the pharmacist is to achieve better health outcomes in all patients. The pharmacy profession in conjunction with medicine, needs to step forward to accept this challenge and make changes for the benefit of patients, society, and providers.

While the pharmacist workforce is well educated (at the doctoral level for the past 40 years) and highly accessible, this widely distributed group of healthcare professionals is vastly underutilized. Recent uptake and desire by patients to have immunizations provided at pharmacies by pharmacists, is a prime example of care that is convenient and cost-effective, yet delivered by another healthcare provider. As pointed out in a 2012 *New York Times* article [6], pharmacists are capable of adjusting medications, ordering and interpreting laboratory tests, and coordinating follow-up care, but state and federal laws complicate this, even though patients prefer the convenience of dealing with pharmacists.

Physicians are also recognizing the underutilized role of the pharmacist. As authored by a physician in the January 28, 2019 *New York Times* article, *The Unsung Role of the Pharmacist in Patient Health* [7] the author contends that in medicine, the focus is far too often solely on the traditional doctor/patient interaction, ignoring other practitioners (such as pharmacists) who come into contact with patients more than physicians, who can help make health care better for all.

Likewise, another physician opined in the 10 October 2018 *Forbes* article, *Can Pharmacists Help Reinvent Primary Care in the United States?* [8] that we need to bring more bright minds into medicine, but we should "not ignore the secret weapon that we already have: pharmacists." He further asserts that in many cases, time-intensive chronic disease management, which currently lies in the hands of doctors and nurse practitioners, can be handed off "to the capable hands of pharmacists-who have a mastery of medication management, as well, as behavior change." In summary, he postulates that by relying on pharmacists and "integrating them in our healthcare delivery models, we can provide better, more affordable, and more effective care to everyone-and potentially alleviate the looming crisis in access to primary care."

A soon to be realized future should be envisioned where pharmacists are embedded in primary care settings as PCPPs. Having a pharmacist involved at the point-of-prescribing (i.e., in clinics) provides tremendous benefits to providers and patients alike including appropriate medication selection, adherence to therapeutic guidelines, conformance with prescription formularies, and soon, precision medicine realized through pharmacogenomics. Benefits include enhanced medication adherence, fewer adverse drug-related events, reduced inappropriate healthcare utilization (e.g., emergency room visits, hospitalizations, office visits), improved clinical outcomes, higher CMS Star Ratings, greater physician and patient satisfaction, and potentially total reduced cost of care.

Additionally, these PCPPs could extend such services in underserved rural and urban areas connected through one or two integrated EHRs, thus allowing for synchronous and asynchronous communications with multiple providers, across multiple health systems as well as with community pharmacist colleagues.

As more and more payment for health services moves from fee-for-service to "value-based", "at-risk", or "pay for performance (P4P)" contracting, it is incumbent that health systems, physicians, and payers need to look at the full complement and shear number of healthcare providers available to meet the needs of society. Certainly, the COVID-19 pandemic of 2020 has brought forward the challenges of an overwhelmed healthcare system and need to embrace all essential healthcare providers, and that embrace needs to include pharmacists. Thought of in another way (from the patient perspective), we need to consider seeing the right patient, by the right provider, in the right place, for the right price, and where appropriate, the use of the right pharmaceutical: "the 5Ps". I subscribe that in fact, pharmacists with physicians can help address these 5Ps in primacy care.

These articles in PHARMACY's Special Issue "Embedded Pharmacists in Primary Care" highlight such advancements of models that have included pharmacists. These contributions span academic medical centers to family medicine training programs in both urban and rural settings as well as performing roles in chronic disease management, comprehensive medication management, and the use of collaborative practice agreements. As Guest Editor to this Special Issue, I hope you enjoy these contributions and that they inspire you to replicate these works by contacting these authors or making your own contribution in the near future!

Be well in this unprecedented times.

References

1. The Complexities of Physician Supply and Demand: Projections from 2018 to 2033. Available online: https://www.aamc.org/system/files/2020-06/stratcomm-aamc-physician-workforce-projections-june-2020.pdf (accessed on 13 August 2020).
2. Bodenheimer, T.; Sinsky, C. From triple to quadruple aim: Care of the patient requires care of the provider. *Ann. Fam. Med.* **2014**, *12*, 573–576. [CrossRef] [PubMed]
3. Improving Patient and Health System Outcomes through Advanced Pharmacy Practice. Available online: https://www.pharmacist.com/improving-patient-and-health-system-outcomes-through-advanced-pharmacy-practice-report-surgeon (accessed on 19 August 2020).
4. Embedding Pharmacists Into the Practice: Collaborate with Pharmacists to Improve Patient Outcomes. Available online: https://edhub.ama-assn.org/steps-forward/module/2702554 (accessed on 19 August 2020).
5. VA Treats Patients' Impatience with Clinical Pharmacists. Available online: https://www.usatoday.com/story/news/2016/10/24/kaiser-va-treats-patients-impatience-clinical-pharmacists/92479132/ (accessed on 19 August 2020).
6. When the Doctor Is Not Needed. Available online: https://www.nytimes.com/2012/12/16/opinion/sunday/when-the-doctor-is-not-needed.html (accessed on 19 August 2020).
7. The Unsung Role of the Pharmacist in Patient Health: Are People Relying too much on the Traditional Doctor/Patient Interaction? Available online: https://www.nytimes.com/2019/01/28/upshot/pharmacists-drugs-health-unsung-role.html (accessed on 19 August 2020).
8. Can Pharmacists Help Reinvent Primary Care in the United States? Available online: https://www.forbes.com/sites/sachinjain/2018/10/10/can-pharmacists-help-reinvent-primary-care-in-the-united-states/#24f3b2e5590b (accessed on 19 August 2020).

Publisher's Note: MDPI stays neutral with regard to jurisdictional claims in published maps and institutional affiliations.

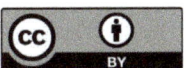

© 2020 by the author. Licensee MDPI, Basel, Switzerland. This article is an open access article distributed under the terms and conditions of the Creative Commons Attribution (CC BY) license (http://creativecommons.org/licenses/by/4.0/).

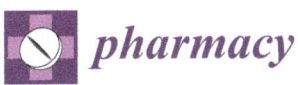

Article

Expansion and Evaluation of Pharmacist Services in Primary Care

Katherine J. Hartkopf [1,*], Kristina M. Heimerl [1], Kayla M. McGowan [1] and Brian G. Arndt [2,3]

1. Department of Pharmacy, University of Wisconsin Health, Madison, WI 53792, USA; kheimerl@uwhealth.org (K.M.H.); kmcgowan@uwhealth.org (K.M.M.)
2. Department of Family Medicine and Community Health, School of Medicine and Public Health, University of Wisconsin, Madison, WI 53706, USA; brian.arndt@fammed.wisc.edu
3. University of Wisconsin Health PATH Collaborative (Primary Care Academics Transforming Healthcare), Madison, WI 53705, USA
* Correspondence: khartkopf@uwhealth.org

Received: 16 June 2020; Accepted: 16 July 2020; Published: 22 July 2020

Abstract: Challenges with primary care access and overextended providers present opportunities for pharmacists as patient care extenders for chronic disease management. The primary objective was to align primary care pharmacist services with organizational priorities and improve patient clinical outcomes. The secondary objective was to develop a technological strategy for service evaluation. An interdisciplinary workgroup developed primary care pharmacist services focused on improving performance measures and supporting the care team in alignment with ongoing population health initiatives. Pharmacist collaborative practice agreements (CPAs) were developed and implemented. An electronic dashboard was developed to capture service outcome measures. Blood pressure control to <140/90 mmHg was achieved in 74.15% of patients who engaged with primary care pharmacists versus 41.53% of eligible patients electing to follow usual care pathways. Appropriate statin use was higher in patients engaged with primary care pharmacists than in eligible patients electing to follow usual care pathways both for diabetes and ischemic vascular disease (12.4% and 2.2% higher, respectively). Seventeen of 54 possible process and outcome measures were identified and incorporated into an electronic dashboard. Primary care pharmacist services improve hypertension control and statin use. Service outcomes can be measured with discrete data from the electronic health record (EHR), and should align with organizational priorities.

Keywords: pharmacist; primary care; collaborative practice agreement; patient care extender; comprehensive medication management; quality improvement; electronic health record; electronic dashboard

1. Introduction

A growing issue in the United States healthcare system is timely access to primary care [1–3]. The population is increasingly comprised of aging individuals with a large number of complex and chronic disease states. Effective, long-term management of these chronic disease states requires careful planning and the establishment of attainable health goals [4–6]. Additionally, shared decision-making should occur between the patient and provider to ensure that appropriate risks and benefits of care are considered. Furthermore, providers are tasked to ensure patients are equipped with the knowledge they need for active involvement in their own care [7]. Differing patient populations require individualized and often complex approaches to care, which consume significant amounts of healthcare resources, including provider time.

In many primary care practices, patient care extenders are under-utilized, which leads to unnecessary burden of clinical and nonclinical activities for the provider. Health systems have started to transition responsibility for lab ordering, patient education, medication titration, refills, prior authorizations, and other similar duties to various lower-cost patient care extenders, at times utilizing disease-specific collaborative practice agreements (CPAs) [8–10]. Innovative use and delegated expanded roles of patient care extenders in primary care are imperative for improved patient outcomes given the ever-rising demand and time constraints on primary care providers [11–14].

Implementation of patient care extenders in a team-based care model has demonstrated enhanced quality of patient care, improved cost-effectiveness, and reduced provider burnout [15–18]. Previously published studies suggest pharmacists practicing in primary care can significantly decrease medication errors, improve health outcomes, and enhance provider satisfaction when functioning as integral members of the patient care team [19–24]. Measuring and reporting service outcomes in a timely manner is vital to implementation and growth of primary care pharmacist roles and has demonstrated, in some cases, improved evidence-based care and patient health outcomes [25,26]. It also allows for rapid quality improvement and alignment of pharmacist resources based on patient population needs. The necessary data to report service outcomes can and should be leveraged from the electronic health record (EHR) and corresponding data warehouses for optimal efficiency and care team visibility.

2. Service Implementation and Evaluation

2.1. Setting

This service was developed at a six-hospital academic medical center (AMC) with 34 primary care clinics and approximately 287,000 medically homed patients. The AMC has residency-focused, community-based, and regional partners in family and internal medicine. Since 2010, the AMC has incorporated efforts to redesign primary care services with specific focus areas of patient-centered care, efficiency, service standardization, and care team member engagement.

2.2. Phase 1 Implementation and Analysis

In 2016, six salaried pharmacist full-time equivalents (FTE) were hired to support further redesign efforts and grow the patient care services offered for comprehensive primary care. Initial pharmacist services were provided to patients with high medication burden ($\geq$13), multiple co-morbid conditions ($\geq$6), and those referred from providers. All initial services were recommendation-based and ultimately required provider approval in order to implement medication changes with patients. As a result, data collection focused on medication interventions completed. Providers were receptive to recommendations from a primary care pharmacist. However, it was challenging to measure value and directly associate pharmacist services with clinical outcomes. Additionally, all data collection was manual, inefficient, and subject to human error. Through partnership with key leaders in the primary care and population health departments at the AMC, the need for pharmacist service revision to better align with organizational population health efforts as well as a dynamic service dashboard was identified.

2.3. Service Revision

The primary objective was to align primary care pharmacist services with organizational priorities and improve patient clinical outcomes. The secondary objective was to develop a direct technological interface with the EHR for pharmacist service evaluation.

A workgroup consisting of the Senior Medical Director of Primary Care, Medical Director of Population Health, Pharmacy Director and Manager of Ambulatory Care Services, and a pharmacy resident convened to redesign primary care pharmacist services. Pharmacist services were developed with information from four sources. Healthcare performance measures, including state-specific quality measures and Accountable Care Organization measures, were assessed to identify opportunities for improvement compared to peer institutions. Proven measures in which pharmacists provide value and improve outcomes were identified using literature searches via PubMed and pharmacy journals. Existing organization-specific primary care workflows and care team roles were considered by the workgroup. Additionally, provider perspectives collected during the intervention-based initial phase of implementation helped inform the service revision proposal.

The top five proposed pharmacy services were identified based on the intersection of organizational need for improvement and published data to support pharmacists improving outcomes in those specific disease states. Additionally, a strategy to expand the existing pharmacist FTE resources to additional primary care clinics and patients was prepared. All aspects of the proposed services aligned with key components of the organization's population health core standards: clear patient inclusion and exclusion criteria, consistent service aspects during initial and follow-up patient outreach, and clear discharge criteria. The proposal specified the patient care pathway if the provider and patient agreed to participate in the pharmacist service. This pathway included the ability for pharmacist identification or provider referral, patient enrollment processes, visit elements and cadence, and discharge back to primary care provider when clinical goals were met or a patient disengaged. Appropriate patient was defined as a patient that required medication titration, and had a history of medication adherence concerns or numerous adverse effects to medications. This was in contrast to usual care processes in which patients were seen in-clinic for scheduled provider visits. The providers were accountable to determine any necessary changes in medication therapy and schedule appropriate follow-up with a provider, nurse, or medical assistant. The resulting pharmacist service proposal was presented to a primary care leadership committee for feedback and ultimate endorsement.

2.4. Phase 2 Implementation

An initial clinic location was identified by the workgroup for implementation of the redesigned pharmacist service. Two primary care pharmacists were assigned to lead the implementation at this location and refine service workflows over a 4-week implementation period. In parallel, CPAs were developed and approved for hypertension and statin medication management to be delegated from providers to trained primary care pharmacists. The structure of the CPAs aligned with organizational requirements and included the following information: patient eligibility criteria, contraindications for use of the CPA, when to consult a provider, treatment goals, documentation requirements, patient follow-up and monitoring, and medications and labs that could be prescribed or ordered by a trained pharmacist.

A team training occurred at the end of the initial clinic implementation period to share the vision and need for service revisions, as well as train all primary care pharmacist team members on the new workflows. When the CPAs were fully approved for implementation, the pharmacists completed targeted team trainings. Each pharmacist was required to participate in a didactic therapeutic review session with a cardiology specialist physician. Additionally, each pharmacist completed two case-based assessments. The first was for the elements contained in the CPA, and the second was a clinical assessment. Pharmacists were required to receive a score of 80% in order to utilize the CPA. In addition to CPA training, all pharmacists pursued board certification in ambulatory care within their first year of hire.

Utilizing a standardized clinic implementation toolkit, the redesigned pharmacist services were implemented at an average of one clinic per month over the span of one year. The clinic implementation toolkit assisted each pharmacist in integrating services into the clinic. Pharmacists were responsible for setting up their patient room, ongoing communication with staff, and sharing successes and barriers with building their patient panels. The EHR integration with clinics included creating a pharmacist schedule, clinic communication pool or in-basket, and pharmacist referral that could be entered by providers.

Continued workgroup meetings identified core process and outcome measures to be tracked and reported to demonstrate service success. A prioritization matrix, a quality improvement tool, was used with the analytics team to identify effort to access and impact of the proposed outcome measures [27,28]. Through engagement and collaboration with analytics and information technology representatives, a service-specific dashboard was developed in external software used throughout the organization. Additionally, a new electronic form was developed within the EHR to capture service process measures in a discrete manner and inform the dashboard. The electronic form was completed by the pharmacist for every patient the pharmacist intended to enroll in services. While the form was open, the pharmacist was providing services to enrolled patients and considered them as part of their panel. Then, upon discharge, the form was completed in its entirety.

This project was determined not to meet the federal definition of research, and the UW-Madison Health Sciences Institutional Review Board certified it as a quality improvement project.

3. Results

The AMC's primary care pharmacist service was redesigned to focus on core services linked to specific clinical outcomes in alignment with selected healthcare performance measure definitions. Hypertension medication management to achieve goal blood pressure <140/90 mmHg, and statin initiation for patients with diabetes or ischemic vascular disease, was completed via CPA to offset provider workload. Individualized patient goals and medication management recommendations presented to patients included assessment of perceived benefits and risks to promote shared decision-making. Pharmacists also remained available for comprehensive medication reviews and care team clinical consults due to provider demand for assisting in care management of complex patients. These services were not directly related to the core services, as they were not linked to specific clinical outcomes. Pharmacists were onsite one to three days per week across 13 of the 34 primary care clinics. When not onsite, services were supported by a centralized triage pharmacist shift.

The CPAs for hypertension and statin services were initiated by provider referral or pharmacist identification via disease state registries. Within the first year of the service revision, 948 patients were identified as eligible for the hypertension service, with 607 (64%) patients engaging in at least one clinical visit with a primary care pharmacist. Clinical measures demonstrated blood pressure was controlled to <140/90 mmHg in 74.15% of patients who engaged with a primary care pharmacist versus 41.53% of eligible patients electing to follow usual care pathways, a difference of 32.6% (Appendix A).

Statin use when indicated was also higher when patients engaged with a primary care pharmacist for an assessment of statin appropriateness, discussed risks versus benefits, and decided whether or not to pursue statin therapy. In the first year of the service revision, 481 patients with diabetes and not on a statin engaged with a primary care pharmacist versus 243 eligible patients who did not engage with the pharmacist. Statin use when indicated was 12.4% higher in the group of patients engaging with the pharmacist service than in those following usual care pathways (82.93% and 70.56%, respectively) (Appendix B). There was also a modest increase in statin use of 2.2% for patients with ischemic vascular disease (98.21% with pharmacists and 96% with usual care) (Appendix C).

Based on a conservative estimate of the lifetime cumulative costs of one fatal cardiovascular event, the first year of the revised services for hypertension management and statin initiation alone produced greater than $1.4 million in cost avoidance [29–32].

In order to develop ongoing service evaluation monitoring, 54 proposed process and outcome measures were evaluated using a prioritization matrix (Appendix D). Seventeen measures were identified with the highest feasibility and greatest impact on service success, and informed the data collection plan. The electronic form developed within the EHR directly linked service patients through an episode of care and discretely tracked the identified process metrics through eight targeted questions. The service-specific dashboard updated daily to provide dynamic information. The dashboard was designed to house individual reports and information that aligned with the data collection plan. Two reports displayed results of the clinical outcomes of service patients and tracked the results over time. Five additional reports linked directly to patient-level data to allow for targeted assessment of outliers and identification of service improvement opportunities. Additionally, two reports emphasized areas of interest from a population health perspective: demographics and mix of patients from our accountable population.

4. Discussion

The medication management responsibilities within this primary care pharmacist service align with the American College of Clinical Pharmacy (ACCP) definition of clinical pharmacists who provide direct patient care [33]. The pharmacists engage in direct assessment and evaluation of patient-specific medication needs; medication selection, initiation, titration, and discontinuation; ongoing monitoring of lab results, side effects, and adherence; and necessary communication with providers when concerns arise. Pharmacists are well trained and prepared to provide this level of patient care, especially in team-based care models [34].

Though this was not a robust, randomized trial of clinical outcomes, this primary care pharmacist service further endorses the positive impact of a pharmacist embedded in the care team. When serving as a patient care extender, the optimal role for a pharmacist involves medication management for chronic disease states. These activities transition workload from providers, and can be directly associated with improving measurable patient health outcomes. As health systems transition to value-based payment models, pharmacists can positively impact quality measures for chronic disease states where medication optimization is key for disease control and prevention of poor outcomes, such as cardiovascular disease [35–38].

There are several limitations of our service evaluation. One notable limitation is patient self-selection bias. Patients who engaged with a pharmacist may be more motivated to improve their health outcomes. Alternatively, patients referred to a pharmacist for medication management may be more complex than patients seen by a nurse or medical assistant through usual care. Randomization would have reduced potential bias; however, it was not pursued due to the quality improvement nature of this work. Another limitation is that several patients followed usual care pathways instead of working with a pharmacist because of capacity. The six pharmacist FTE are not able to reach all patients, so targeted efforts and patient prioritization is key.

An additional key limitation of our year one evaluation and dashboard development has been an inability to capture the primary care pharmacist service impact of comprehensive medication reviews for patients at risk of readmission. This, in addition to service impact on unintended hospitalizations, will be considered for future service evaluation.

While healthcare performance measures are beneficial to benchmark success, they can be restrictive and may not fully reflect the service impact. Given the inclusion of shared decision-making between pharmacist and patient, there are patients who believe the possible benefit does not outweigh the potential risk and the resulting outcome does not positively align with the designated performance measure.

The service redesign efforts and processes help guide others through a process of evaluating organizational need and population health standards to align services provided by pharmacists in primary care. It also demonstrates identification of a systematic data collection plan that will interface with discrete information available through the EHR to inform a dashboard with meaningful, dynamic, and timely data. All process and clinical results provided in this year-one evaluation were extracted directly from the service dashboard, required no manipulation, and continue to be updated daily. The data can be utilized for ongoing quality improvement and to support realignment and growth of services to meet changing organizational needs in alignment with prior research [39,40].

5. Conclusions

There is an opportunity in the primary care setting to introduce new clinical pharmacist services, along with an effort to reallocate medication management activities from providers, while aligning with organizational priorities such as improved hypertension control and statin use. Clear definition of pharmacist service measures and a direct interface with discrete data from the EHR allows for optimal evaluation of both clinical and operational impacts.

Author Contributions: Each author made substantial contributions to the work including, conceptualization, K.J.H., K.M.H., K.M.M. and B.G.A.; methodology, K.J.H. and K.M.H.; software, K.J.H.; validation, K.M.H. and K.M.M.; formal analysis, K.J.H.; investigation, K.J.H.; resources, K.J.H.; data curation, K.J.H.; writing—original draft preparation, K.J.H. and K.M.H.; writing—review and editing, K.M.M. and B.G.A.; visualization, K.M.H.; supervision, K.J.H. and B.G.A.; project administration, K.J.H. and K.M.H. All authors have read and agreed to the published version of the manuscript.

Funding: This research received no external funding.

Acknowledgments: The authors acknowledge the contribution of Matthew Anderson and Jeffrey Huebner for their support and guidance throughout service redesign.

Conflicts of Interest: The authors declare no conflict of interest.

Appendix A

Table A1. Blood Pressure Control.

		Blood Pressure Control (n = 948)		
Year	Month	% Controlled RPh (n = 607)	% Controlled Non-RPh (n = 341)	(% Controlled RPh)– (% Controlled Non-RPh)
2017	Jun	70.7	60.66	10.0
	Jul	71.67	59.78	11.9
	Aug	67.04	58.60	8.4
	Sept	67.13	54.23	12.9
	Oct	35.78	52.36	13.4
	Nov	63.61	50.53	13.1
	Dec	61.04	44.16	16.9
2018	Jan	63.59	44.39	19.2
	Feb	63.43	42.59	20.8
	Mar	64.06	43.66	20.2
	Apr	66.3	40.08	26.2
	May	70.41	40.98	29.4
	Jun	74.15	41.53	32.6
	Jul	73.6	41.04	32.6
	Aug	73.98	43.49	30.8

Appendix B

Table A2. Statin Use—Diabetes.

		Statin Use in Patients with Diabetes (n = 724)		
Year	Month	% Statins RPh (n = 481)	% Statins Non-RPh (n = 243)	(% Statins RPh)– (% Statins Non-RPh)
2017	Jun	71.3	59.75	11.6
	Jul	72.31	59.26	13.1
	Aug	72.36	58.18	14.2
	Sept	72.81	57.99	14.8
	Oct	71.94	59.77	12.2
	Nov	73.98	61.33	12.7
	Dec	75.86	62.64	13.2
2018	Jan	76.86	63.89	13.0
	Feb	77.27	64.25	13.0
	Mar	78.75	66.84	11.9
	Apr	79.83	66.56	13.2
	May	81.74	68.72	13.0
	Jun	82.93	70.56	12.4
	Jul	83.02	69.90	13.1
	Aug	83.24	70	13.2

Appendix C

Table A3. Statin Use—Ischemic Vascular Disease.

Year	Month	Statin Use in Patients with IVD (n = 278)		
		% Statins RPh (n = 195)	% Statins Non-RPh (n = 83)	(% Statins RPh)– (% Statins Non-RPh)
2017	Jun	93.26	86.05	7.2
	Jul	93.41	84.09	9.3
	Aug	93.41	84.09	9.3
	Sept	93.41	85.71	7.7
	Oct	93.62	88.37	5.3
	Nov	94.62	90.91	3.7
	Dec	95.83	89.58	6.3
2018	Jan	95.05	89.8	5.3
	Feb	96.04	89.58	6.5
	Mar	96.15	93.33	2.8
	Apr	96.49	93.48	3.0
	May	97.32	93.75	3.6
	Jun	98.21	96	2.2
	Jul	99.07	96	3.1
	Aug	99.12	96.23	2.9

Appendix D

Table A4. Measure Prioritization.

Priority	Measure
5–11	Wisconsin Collaborative for Healthcare Quality Outcomes a. Hypertension: Controlling high blood pressure b. Hypertension: Daily aspirin or other antiplatelet for diabetes patients c. Diabetes: Statin use d. Diabetes: Daily aspirin or other antiplatelet for diabetes patients e. Ischemic vascular disease (IVD): Blood pressure control f. Ischemic vascular disease (IVD): Daily aspirin or other antiplatelet unless contraindicated g. Ischemic vascular disease (IVD): Statin use
1–4	Service Success a. Patient dropout rate b. Reason for service graduation/discontinuation c. Length of time spent in service d. Number of patients enrolled
13–14	Readmission a. Readmission reduction (30 and 90 day) b. Cost avoidance of potential readmissions
16–17	Satisfaction Patient satisfaction with pharmacist services Provider satisfaction with pharmacist services
12	Patients per pharmacist per hour
15	Adherence to the CPAs for hypertension and lipids

References

1. American College of Physicians. *How is a Shortage of Primary Care Physicians Affecting the Quality and Cost of Medical Care? A Comprehensive Evidence Review*; American College of Physicians: Philadelphia, PA, USA, 2008.
2. Cheung, P.T.; Wiler, J.L.; Lowe, R.A.; Ginde, A.A. National study of barriers to timely primary care and emergency department utilization among Medicaid beneficiaries. *Ann. Emerg. Med.* **2012**, *60*, 4–10.e2. [CrossRef]
3. Kravet, S.J.; Shore, A.D.; Miller, R.; Green, G.B.; Kolodner, K.; Wright, S.M. Health care utilization and the proportion of primary care physicians. *Am. J. Med.* **2008**, *121*, 142–148. [CrossRef] [PubMed]
4. Bayliss, E.A.; Ellis, J.L.; Steiner, J.F.; Bayliss, E.A.; Ellis, J.L.; Steiner, J.F. Barriers to self-management and quality-of-life outcomes in seniors with multimorbidities. *Ann. Fam. Med.* **2007**, *5*, 395–402. [CrossRef] [PubMed]
5. McGilton, K.S.; Vellani, S.; Yeung, L.; Chishtie, J.; Commisso, E.; Ploeg, J.; Andrew, M.K.; Ayala, A.P.; Gray, M.; Morgan, D.; et al. Identifying and understanding the health and social care needs of older adults with multiple chronic conditions and their caregivers: A scoping review. *BMC Geriatr.* **2018**, *18*, 231. [CrossRef] [PubMed]
6. Smith, S.M.; O'Kelly, S.; O'Dowd, T. GPs' and pharmacists' experiences of managing multimorbidity: A 'Pandora's box. *Br. J. Gen. Pract.* **2010**, *60*, e285–e294. [CrossRef] [PubMed]
7. Barrett, B.; Ricco, J.; Wallace, M.; Kiefer, D.; Rakel, D. Communicating statin evidence to support shared decision-making. *BMC Fam. Pract.* **2016**, *17*, 41. [CrossRef]
8. Bodenheimer, T.; Ghorob, A.; Willard-Grace, R.; Grumbach, K. The 10 building blocks of high-performing primary care. *Ann. Fam. Med.* **2014**, *12*, 166–171. [CrossRef]
9. Lee, T.H. Care redesign—A path forward for providers. *N. Engl. J. Med.* **2012**, *367*, 466–472. [CrossRef]
10. Yarnall, K.S.; Østbye, T.; Krause, K.M.; Pollak, K.I.; Gradison, M.; Michener, J.L. Family physicians as team leaders: "time" to share the care. *Prev. Chronic Dis.* **2009**, *6*, A59.
11. Bodenheimer, T.; Sinsky, C. From triple to quadruple aim: Care of the patient requires care of the provider. *Ann. Fam. Med.* **2014**, *12*, 573–576. [CrossRef]
12. Dyrbye, L.N.; Shanafelt, T.D.; Sinsky, C.A.; Cipriano, P.F.; Bhatt, J.; Ommaya, A.; West, C.P.; Meyers, D. Burnout among health care professionals. A call to explore and address this underrecognized threat to safe, high-quality care. *Natl. Acad. Med.* **2017**, 1–11. [CrossRef]
13. Welp, A.; Meier, L.L.; Manser, T. Emotional exhaustion and workload predict clinician-rated and objective patient safety. *Front Psychol.* **2015**, *5*, 1–13. [CrossRef] [PubMed]
14. Write, A.A.; Katz, I.T. Beyond burnout- redesigning care to restore meaning and sanity for physicians. *N. Engl. J. Med.* **2018**, *378*, 309–311.
15. AMA STEPSforward. *Implementing Team-Based Care to Increase Practice Efficiency*; American Medical Association: Chicago, IL, USA, 2017; Available online: https://edhub.ama-assn.org/steps-forward (accessed on 4 June 2019).
16. Schectman, G.; Wolff, N.; Byrd, J.C.; Hiatt, J.G.; Hartz, A. Physician extenders for cost-effective management of hypercholesterolemia. *J. Gen. Intern. Med.* **1996**, *11*, 277–286. [CrossRef] [PubMed]
17. Sinsky, C.A.; Bodenheimer, T. Powering-Up Primary Care Teams: Advanced Team Care with In-Room Support. *Ann. Fam. Med.* **2019**, *17*, 367–371. [CrossRef] [PubMed]
18. Wagner, E.H.; Flinter, M.; Hsu, C.; Cromp, D.; Austin, B.T.; Etz, R.; Crabtree, B.F.; Ladden, M.D. Effective team-based primary care: Observations from innovative practices. *BMC Fam. Pract.* **2017**, *18*, 1–13. [CrossRef] [PubMed]
19. Funk, K.A.; Pestka, D.L.; McClurg, M.T.; Carroll, J.K.; Sorensen, T.D. Primary care providers believe that comprehensive medication management improves their work-life. *J. Am. Board Fam. Med.* **2019**, *32*, 462–473. [CrossRef]
20. Ip, E.J.; Shah, B.M.; Yu, J.; Chan, J.; Nguyen, L.T.; Bhatt, D.C. Enhancing diabetes care by adding a pharmacist to the primary care team. *Am. J. Health Syst. Pharm.* **2017**, *70*, 877–886. [CrossRef]
21. Moreno, G.; Lonowski, S.; Fu, J.; Chon, J.S.; Whitmire, N.; Vasquez, C.; Skootsky, S.A.; Bell, D.S.; Maranon, R.; Mangione, C.M. Physician experiences with clinical pharmacists in primary care teams. *J. Am. Pharm. Assoc.* **2017**, *57*, 686–691. [CrossRef]
22. Riggins, S.R.; Abode, A.M.; Holland, C.R.; Rhodes, L.A.; Marciniak, M.W. Assessing care team perspectives on integration of a community pharmacist into an ambulatory care practice. *J. Am. Pharm. Assoc.* **2019**. [CrossRef]

23. Smith, M.; Bates, D.W.; Bodenheimer, T.; Cleary, P.D. Why pharmacists belong in the medical home. *Health Aff.* **2010**, *29*, 906–913. [CrossRef] [PubMed]
24. Truong, H.; Kroehl, M.E.; Lewis, C.; Pettigrew, R.; Bennett, M.; Saseen, J.J.; Trinkley, K.E. Clinical pharmacists in primary care: Provider satisfaction and perceived impact on quality of care provided. *SAGE Open Med.* **2017**. [CrossRef] [PubMed]
25. Ahern, D.K.; Stinson, L.J.; Uebelacker, L.A.; Wroblewski, J.P.; McMurray, J.H.; Eaton, C.B. E-health blood pressure control program. *J. Med. Pract. Manag.* **2012**, *28*, 91–100.
26. McMenamin, J.; Nicholson, R.; Leech, K. Patient Dashboard: The use of a colour-coded computerised clinical reminder in Whanganui regional general practices. *J. Prim. Health Care* **2011**, *3*, 307–310. [CrossRef]
27. Breyfogle, F. *Implementing Six Sigma*, 2nd ed.; John Wiley: Hoboken, NJ, USA, 2003.
28. Brassard, M. *The Six Sigma Memory Jogger II*, 1st ed.; Goal QPC: Salem, NH, USA, 2002.
29. Baient, C.; Keech, A.; Kearney, P.M.; Blackwell, L.; Buck, G.; Pollicino, C.; Kirby, A.; Sourjina, T.; Peto, R.; Collins, R.; et al. Efficacy and safety of cholesterol-lowering treatment: Prospective meta-analysis of data from 90,056 participants in 14 randomised trials of statins. *Lancet* **2005**, *366*, 1267–1278.
30. Benjamin, E.J.; Blaha, M.J.; Chiuve, S.E.; Cushman, M.; Das, S.R.; Deo, R.; de Ferranti, S.D.; Floyd, J.; Fornage, M.; Gillespie, C.; et al. Heart disease and stroke statistics—2017 update: A report from the American Heart Association. *Circulation* **2017**, *125*, e229–e445. [CrossRef]
31. Law, M.R.; Morris, J.K.; Wald, N.J. Use of blood pressure lowering drugs in the prevention of cardiovascular disease: Meta-analysis of 147 randomised trials in the context of expectations from prospective epidemiological studies. *Br. Med. J.* **2009**, *383*, 1665. [CrossRef]
32. O'Sullivan, A.K.; Rubin, J.; Nyambose, J.; Kuznik, A.; Cohen, D.; Thompson, D. Cost estimation of cardiovascular disease events in the US. *Pharmacoeconomics* **2011**, *29*, 693–704. [CrossRef]
33. American College of Clinical Pharmacy (ACCP). Board of Regents commentary. Qualifications of pharmacists who provide direct patient care: Perspectives on the need for residency training and board certification. *Pharmacotherapy* **2013**, *33*. [CrossRef]
34. McBane, S.E.; Dopp, A.L.; Abe, A.; Benavides, S.; Chester, E.A.; Dixon, D.L.; Dunn, M.; Johnson, M.D.; Nigro, S.J.; Rothrock-Christian, T.; et al. Collaborative drug therapy management and comprehensive medication management—2015. *Pharmacotherapy* **2015**, *35*, e39–e50.
35. Moore, R.; Nickerson-Troy, J.; Morse, K.; Finley, K. Enhancing Pharmacy Services in a Primary Care Setting to Help Providers Improve Quality Performance Measures. *Am. J. Health Syst. Pharm.* **2019**, *76*, 1460–1461. [CrossRef] [PubMed]
36. Sinclair, J.; Santoso Bentley, O.; Abubakar, A.; Marciniak, M.W. Impact of a Pharmacist in Improving Quality Measures That Affect Payments to Physicians. *J. Am. Pharm. Assoc.* **2019**, *59*, S85–S90. [CrossRef] [PubMed]
37. Awdishu, L.; Singh, R.F.; Saunders, I.; Yam, F.K.; Hirsch, J.D.; Lorentz, S.; Atayee, R.S.; Ma, J.D.; Tsunoda, S.M.; Namba, J.; et al. Advancing Pharmacist Collaborative Care within Academic Health Systems. *Pharmacy* **2019**, *7*, 142. [CrossRef] [PubMed]
38. Dunn, S.P.; Birtcher, K.K.; Beavers, C.J.; Baker, W.L.; Brouse, S.D.; Page, R.L., 2nd; Bittner, V.; Walsh, M.N. The Role of the Clinical Pharmacist in the Care of Patients with Cardiovascular Disease. *J. Am. Coll. Cardiol.* **2015**, *66*, 2129–2139. [CrossRef] [PubMed]
39. Wilbanks, B.A.; Langford, P.A. A review of dashboards for data analytics in nursing. *Comput. Inform. Nurs.* **2014**, *32*, 545–549. [CrossRef] [PubMed]
40. Frith, K.H.; Anderson, F.; Sewell, J.P. Assessing and selecting data for a nursing services dashboard. *J. Nurs. Adm.* **2010**, *40*, 10–16. [CrossRef]

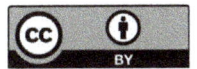

© 2020 by the authors. Licensee MDPI, Basel, Switzerland. This article is an open access article distributed under the terms and conditions of the Creative Commons Attribution (CC BY) license (http://creativecommons.org/licenses/by/4.0/).

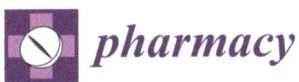

Article

How a State Measures Up: Ambulatory Care Pharmacists' Perception of Practice Management Systems for Comprehensive Medication Management in Utah

Kyle Turner [1,2,*], Alan Abbinanti [1], Bradly Winter [3], Benjamin Berrett [2], Jeff Olson [3] and Nicholas Cox [1,2]

1. Department of Pharmacotherapy, College of Pharmacy, University of Utah, Salt Lake City, UT 84112, USA; alan.abbinanti@pharm.utah.edu (A.A.); nicholas.cox@pharm.utah.edu (N.C.)
2. University of Utah Health, Salt Lake City, UT 84132, USA; golden.berrett@hsc.utah.edu
3. Intermountain Pharmacy Services, Intermountain Health Care, Salt Lake City, UT 84102, USA; bradly.winter@imail.org (B.W.); jeff.olson@imail.org (J.O.)
* Correspondence: kyle.turner@pharm.utah.edu; Tel.: +1-801-587-7728

Received: 17 June 2020; Accepted: 25 July 2020; Published: 1 August 2020

Abstract: Comprehensive medication management (CMM) is a patient-centered standard of care that ensures a patient's medications are optimized. The CMM Practice Management Assessment Tool (PMAT) is a tool to assess areas of CMM practice management. The purpose of this project was to assess the state of CMM practice management based on clinical pharmacist perception for two health systems in the state of Utah, and to identify areas of excellence and/or improvement utilizing a novel method for PMAT analysis. The PMAT was distributed to all primary care-focused ambulatory care pharmacists employed by University of Utah Health (U of U Health) and Intermountain Healthcare (Intermountain). Ordinal responses were assigned to three possible categories of CMM support (High, Indifferent, and Low). Ten surveys were completed from U of U Health, and nine were completed from Intermountain. Thirty-two of the 86 survey questions resulted in a high level of support, and 25 questions resulted in a low level of support from the majority of respondents. Statistically significant differences between the institutions were found for 18 questions. The utilization of the PMAT within two Utah health systems highlighted areas of excellence and improvement and demonstrates a unique method for analysis of PMAT results.

Keywords: comprehensive medications management; practice management; ambulatory care; primary care; clinical pharmacy

1. Introduction

Comprehensive Medication Manage (CMM) is a patient-centered care process that ensures each patient's medications are individually assessed to determine that each medication is indicated for a particular condition, is effective for the medical condition and achieving defined goals, is safe given the comorbidities and other medications being taken, and that the patient is able to take the medication as intended and adhere to the prescribed regimen [1,2]. CMM consists of three core elements: philosophy of practice, patient care process, and practice management system [1,2]. CMM has been shown to significantly improve clinical, financial, and humanistic outcomes when implemented [3–8]. Due to CMM's beneficial impact on key outcomes, two institutions in the state of Utah—University of Utah Health (U of U Health) [9] and Intermountain Healthcare (Intermountain)—sought to implement CMM within primary care clinics at each health system. Recognizing that a functional practice management system was essential to effective implementation of CMM [10], the two health systems partnered to assess and compare results for insight into improvement strategies.

To aid the implementation of CMM, the Utah Alliance of Ambulatory Pharmacists (UAAP) was created as a practice advancement and advocacy learning collaborative to represent the voice of pharmacists in ambulatory care across the state. Representatives from U of U Health and Intermountain were founding members of UAAP. Utilizing the knowledge and relationships in UAAP, the two institutions partnered to improve their practice management systems in hopes of learning from one another and disseminating that learning to other members of UAAP. Inherent in this collaborative effort was the ultimate goal of practice management improvement within each organization, to gain the resources and essential elements of CMM needed to advance practice within the state.

Efforts to implement CMM through collaboration in UAAP centered on the work of the CMM in Primary Care Research Team [11,12], with the selection of the Practice Management Assessment Tool (PMAT) [12] as the instrument to determine the current state of practice management systems at the two institutions. The PMAT is a relatively new tool developed and validated by the University of Minnesota's Department of Pharmaceutical Care and Health Systems to assess the level of support for CMM within an organization [12]. Due to its recent development, the use of the PMAT is limited and few articles have been published on its application in a novel environment. The purpose of this project was to assess the state of CMM practice management based on clinical pharmacist perception for two health systems in the state of Utah and to identify areas of excellence and/or improvement utilizing a novel method for PMAT analysis.

2. Methods

The PMAT consists of 86 questions regarding CMM support in various pharmacy practice areas, including 5 essential domains: Organizational Support, Care Team Engagement, Care Delivery Processes, CMM Program Evaluation, and Ensuring Quality Care. The first 5 questions use a Likert scale (from 1 to 10) to assess the 5 domains of CMM practice management's performance and feasibility. The remaining 81 questions used a mix of categorical rankings to further assess the 5 domains, as well as essential components of CMM practice management. For example, a question asked, "Which of the following statements is most true for your practice site regarding availability of patient care space?". Possible responses were "There is not a designated space and it is difficult to find space", "There is not a designated space but it is not difficult to find space", "There is a designated space", "There are two or more designated spaces". The PMAT was distributed to all primary care pharmacists within the two institutions to assess each individual practice. If multiple pharmacists or a pharmacy technician practiced within the site, one version of the PMAT was completed after input and collaboration from all involved.

Comparisons between questions or collaborating institutions could not be made using the native PMAT due to differing scales used for multiple questions. To overcome this issue, we created a uniform ordinal answer scale for all questions thus allowing for comparisons and determination of statistical differences. Each question's possible responses were converted into an ordinal response of three possible groups: High, Indifferent, and Low support. Group categorization decisions were reviewed by a committee of 5 independent non-affiliated instigators who determined what possible responses were considered High, Indifferent, and Low for each individual question and its respective answer choices (See Supplementary Materials). For questions that only consisted of two possible answer choices, the Indifferent support category was excluded as a possible categorization. For questions that consisted of a "select all that apply" answer set, a range of selected choices was designated for each category (ex. High = 8–12, Indifferent = 4–7, Low = 0–3). For instance, in the above example question and answer set, responses indicating two or more spaces were considered High, having a dedicated space was indifferent and the two options stating there was not a dedicated space were considered Low, regardless if it was difficult to find spare or not. Each question was reviewed individually to create a unique categorization of its answers for High, Indifferent, and Low.

Surveys were distributed and collected via a paper copy in mandatory monthly meetings for clinical pharmacists at U of U Health, and via a Qualtrics survey at Intermountain. After surveys were completed, results were manually converted to the designated support categories. Comparisons between institutions were made using a Fischer exact test, due to a small sample size, and by comparing the number of High Support responses to non-High Support responses (i.e., Indifferent Support + Low Support)., and Low Support responses to non-Low Support responses (i.e., High Support + Indifferent Support). This was done to better identify differences in High and Low support by combining the Indifferent category with the opposite category being evaluated, and highlight areas of strength and opportunity between the institutions.

3. Results

All primary care pharmacy teams were given the PMAT and a 100% response rate was achieved, with a total of ten surveys completed from U of U Health and nine from Intermountain. Of the first five general questions regarding the five domains of CMM practice management, only one question demonstrated High Support responses from the majority of respondents (50% or more), specifically the feasibility of ensuring quality care. None of the first five general questions demonstrated Low Support from the majority of respondents (50% or more) or showed a statistically significant difference between the two institutions. The results are summarized in Table 1.

Table 1. Results of questions with High Support from the majority of respondents (50% or more).

PMAT Questions	Responses Categorized as High Support (%)
Organizational Support	
Which of the following statements is most true for your practice site regarding availability of patient care space?	58%
… availability of non-patient care space?	68%
… privacy of space?	74%
… size of space?	89%
… care space equipment?	89%
… clinical pharmacy leadership?	63%
Care Team Engagement	
… direct provider referrals?	63%
… placing new referrals to other care team members?	84%
… the ability to order labs?	95%
… the ability to order durable medical equipment? (e.g., blood pressure cuff)	68%
… point-of-care testing?	79%
Care Delivery Processes	
… patient identification for CMM services?	79%
… non-provider referrals?	74%

Table 1. Cont.

PMAT Questions	Responses Categorized as High Support (%)
... generated quality care lists?	79%
... scheduling in EHR?	79%
... automatic appointment reminders?	68%
... scheduling assistance? (Clinic level scheduling)	74%
... scheduling assistance? (Reminder calls)	74%
... scheduling assistance? (Ensuring referrals get scheduled)	63%
... scheduling assistance? (Ensuring follow-up appointments get scheduled)	68%
... outreach? (Outbound calling)	53%
... system access to the documentation system?	95%
... double documentation?	53%
... completion of documentation?	58%
... documentation of Medication Therapy Problems (MTPs)?	63%
... documentation improvement initiatives?	74%
... the requirement of a physician's co-signature?	100%
CMM Program Evaluation	
... the identification of Medication Therapy Problems (MTPs)?	63%
... aggregated-level data extraction?	58%
Ensuring Consistent and Quality Care	
On a scale of 0–10, with 10 being most feasible, how would you rate the feasibility of improving ensuring consistent and quality care in your CMM practice?	58%
... the process to ensure pharmacists are providing consistent and quality care?	53%
... the process to ensure notes have met documentation requirements?	74%

Thirty-two of the 86 survey questions resulted in a High level of support from the majority of respondents (50% or more) from both institutions (see Table 1). Key questions that demonstrated High levels of support include questions about adequate space for CMM activities, support from referrals, point of care testing, availability of equipment, support personnel, and scheduling and documentation. Twenty-five questions resulted in a Low level of support from the majority of respondents (50% or more) from both institutions (see Table 2). Key questions that demonstrated Low levels of support include questions about executive leadership support, collaborative care visits, image ordering, rooming and intake of patients, dedicated support personnel, and patient satisfaction feedback.

Table 2. Results of questions with Low Support from the majority of respondents (50% or more).

PMAT Questions	Responses Categorized as Low Support (%)
Organizational Support	
… clinic leadership?	53%
… executive leadership?	89%
Care Team Engagement	
… collaborative visits?	63%
… the presence of a champion?	58%
… orienting new care team members?	74%
… the ability to order imaging? (e.g., DXA * scan)	95%
… rooming patients?	84%
… the taking of vitals for patients during appointments?	79%
… billing and coding?	84%
… dedicated support personnel? (e.g., MA **, LPN ***)	58%
Care Delivery Processes	
… payer referrals?	84%
… appointment management? (check all that apply)	68%
… outreach? (Other mailings (e.g., brochure))	83%
… efficiency of inputting notes? (check all that apply)	65%
CMM Program Evaluation	
… the resolution of MTPs?	53%
… revenue generation?	53%
… estimated cost savings?	63%
… descriptive measures?	58%
… patient satisfaction?	100%
… patient-level data extraction?	53%
Ensuring Consistent and Quality Care	
… the training process for CMM philosophy of practice?	68%
… the training process for CMM patient care process?	58%
… the training process for CMM practice management?	58%
… for training?	63%
… the use of quality assurance processes for improvement?	53%

* Dual-energy X-ray absorptiometry; ** Medical Assistant; *** Licensed Practical Nurse.

In comparing the two institutions, U of U Health showed statistically higher support than Intermountain in eight questions ($p \leq 0.0325$), while Intermountain showed statistically higher CMM support in one question ($p = 0.0055$) (see Table 3). U of U Health showed higher support in areas of scheduling, point of care testing, support staff, and referrals, while Intermountain showed higher support for double documentation of visits. When evaluating Low support areas, U of U Health showed lower support in one question ($p = 0.0055$) regarding double documentation, while Intermountain showed lower support in eight questions ($p \leq 0.0325$) about provider/pharmacist team satisfaction, data collection, and overall consistency (See Table 4).

Table 3. Statistically significant results of questions illustrating High Support.

PMAT Questions	Responses Considered High UofU * (%)	Responses Considered High IHC ** (%)	p-Value
… direct provider referrals?	90%	33%	0.0198
… point-of-care testing?	100%	56%	0.0325
… dedicated support personnel? (e.g., MA ***, LPN ****)	50%	0%	0.0325
… patient identification for CMM services?	100%	56%	0.0325
… scheduling in EHR?	100%	56%	0.0325
… scheduling assistance? (Centralized scheduling)	80%	11%	0.0055
… scheduling assistance? (Preparing patients for visit expectations)	80%	11%	0.0055
… scheduling assistance? (Ensuring referrals get scheduled)	100%	22%	0.0007
… double documentation?	20%	89%	0.0055
Totals	48%	31%	<0.00001

Note: Only questions with statistically significant differences were included. * University of Utah Health Care; ** Intermountain Health Care; *** Medical Assistant; **** Licensed Practical Nurse.

Table 4. Statistically significant results of questions illustrating Low Support.

PMAT Questions	Responses Considered Low UofU (%)	Responses Considered Low IHC (%)	p-Value
… scheduling assistance? (Centralized scheduling)	20%	78%	0.023
… double documentation?	80%	11%	0.0055
… clinical markers? (e.g., ACT * score, blood pressure, A1C **)	0%	56%	0.0108
… revenue generation?	10%	100%	0.0001
… estimated cost savings?	30%	100%	0.0031
… provider/team satisfaction?	0%	67%	0.0108
… the use of collected CMM data? (select all that apply)	0%	78%	0.0007
… the reporting of CMM data? (select all that apply)	0%	100%	0
… the process to ensure pharmacists are providing consistent and quality care?	0%	44%	0.0325
Totals	27%	46%	<0.00001

Note: Only questions with statistically significant differences were included; * Asthma Control Test; ** Percent Glycated Hemoglobin (Hemoglobin A1C).

4. Discussion

To our knowledge, this is the first paper published documenting the administration and analysis of the PMAT within health system primary care practices with novel CMM implementation and can be used to demonstrate its utility in assessing, planning for, and obtaining essential CMM resources. The initial utilization of the PMAT, and subsequent methodology for analyzing the results, uncovered several areas of excellence and improvement for each institution.

Areas of excellence include adequate space for CMM activities, referrals, point of care testing, equipment availability, support personnel, scheduling, and documentation. Areas where improvement is needed included rooming of patients, collaborative visits, dedicated support personnel, and a greater emphasis on patient feedback. The results will serve as a benchmark for both institutions and inform collaboration to advance practice. We anticipate that these results will be compared against future assessments utilizing the PMAT to determine progress in addressing identified areas for improvement. As a statewide ambulatory care collaborative, UAAP will use the results of this analysis to determine where state-level practice advancements are needed and lobby both institutional and government stakeholders for adequate resources.

Beyond collaboration, the utilization of the PMAT has created organizational and administrative changes within these institutions. For example, U of U Health has built the leadership structure for primary care services based on the five categories of CMM practice management and has identified stewards for the advancement of these areas. Moreover, Intermountain has begun pilot programs aimed at improving pharmacist satisfaction and modified certain data collection strategies.

The strengths of this paper include publication on the administration and analysis of the PMAT and offers a unique methodology for analyzing answers and comparing sites/institutions from the PMAT, a tool that was not initially designed for such investigation. This methodology can be used by other institutions that intend to utilize the PMAT to evaluate their CMM support.

Limitations include a small sample size making it difficult to meet power and detect differences between institutions for many questions. Another limitation of this paper is that the survey was utilized by only two health systems in one state. Further, variation in CMM practice history and institutional structure and priorities exist between the health systems that may account for differences in practice management systems.

This project highlights areas of excellence within Utah and multiple opportunities for improvement in practice management systems related to CMM implementation. Overall, health systems in Utah generally allow for High levels of practice through support for CMM. The results will be used to prioritize efforts to improve CMM implementation within healthcare institutions and within the state and will provide information about potential pitfalls in CMM practice management. It will also provide information on possible methods for future implementation and analysis of the PMAT to other healthcare systems nationally, allowing for greater development and advancement of CMM and enhanced collaboration and standardization of CMM practices.

5. Conclusions

The utilization of the PMAT within two Utah health systems highlighted areas of excellence and improvement within each institution and demonstrated a unique method for analysis of PMAT results. Results can be used by other systems and practices in their CMM implementation with regard to practice management. Overall, health systems in Utah generally allow for high levels of practice through support for CMM. The results will be used to prioritize efforts to improve CMM implementation through collaboration within both healthcare systems and will provide information to other healthcare systems nationally about potential pitfalls in CMM practice management.

Supplementary Materials: The following are available online at http://www.mdpi.com/2226-4787/8/3/136/s1.

Author Contributions: K.T.: Writing—conceptualization, original draft preparation, review and editing, supervision. K.T. was the lead in overseeing the project and creation of the manuscript. A.A.: Software, formal analysis, validation, writing—original draft preparation. A.A. worked on the data analysis and manuscript preparation. B.W.: Resource, data curation, writing—review and editing. B.W. served as the lead contact for Intermountain and was responsible for seeing that the survey was administered to system pharmacists. He engaged in the review and editing of the manuscript. B.B.: Project administration, writing—review and editing. B.B. supervises the primary care pharmacists at University of Utah Health and was instrumental in the design and execution of the project. He engaged in the review and editing of the manuscript. J.O.: Project administration, writing—review and editing. J.O. supervises the primary care pharmacists at Intermountain and was instrumental in the design and execution of the project. He engaged in the review and editing of the manuscript. N.C.: Supervision, formal analysis, writing—review and editing. N.C. provided supervision to the data analysis and was key in the expanding of the project to multiple sites, project administration, writing—review and editing. He engaged in the review and editing of the manuscript. All authors have read and agreed to the published version of the manuscript.

Funding: This research received no external funding.

Acknowledgments: We appreciate the efforts of the primary care pharmacists in each health system who contributed to this project.

Conflicts of Interest: The authors declare no conflicts of interest.

References

1. The Patient Care Process for Delivering Comprehensive Medication Management (CMM): Optimizing Medication Use in Patient-Centered, Team-Based Care Settings. CMM in Primary Care Research Team. Available online: https://www.accp.com/docs/positions/misc/CMM_Care_Process.pdf (accessed on 24 July 2020).
2. McInnis, T.; Webb, E.; Strand, L. *Patient Centered Primary Care Collaborative (PCPCC). The Patient Centered Medical Home: Integrating Comprehensive Medication Management to Optimize Patient Outcomes Resource Guide*, 2nd ed.; PCPCC: Washington, DC, USA, 2012. Available online: www.pcpcc.org/sites/default/files/media/medmanagement.pdf (accessed on 24 July 2020).
3. Brummel, A.; Carlson, A.M. Comprehensive Medication Management and Medication Adherence for Chronic Conditions. *JMCP* **2016**, *1*, 56–62. [CrossRef]
4. Isetts, B.J.; Brown, L.M.; Schondelmeyer, S.W.; Lenarz, L.A. Quality assessment of a collaborative approach for decreasing drug-related morbidity and achieving therapeutic goals. *Arch. Intern. Med.* **2003**, *163*, 1813–1820. [CrossRef]
5. Rao, D.; Gilbert, A.; Strand, L.M.; Cipolle, R.J. Drug therapy problems found in ambulatory patient populations in Minnesota and South Australia. *Pharm. World Sci.* **2007**, *29*, 647–654. [CrossRef] [PubMed]
6. Isetts, B.J.; Schondelmeyer, S.W.; Artz, M.B.; Lenarz, L.A.; Heaton, A.H.; Wadd, W.B.; Brown, L.M.; Cipolle, R.J. Clinical and economic outcomes of medication therapy management services: The Minnesota experience. *J. Am. Pharm. Assoc.* **2008**, *48*, 203–211. [CrossRef] [PubMed]
7. de Oliveira, D.R.; Brummel, A.R.; Miller, D.B. Medication therapy management: 10 years of experience in a large integrated health care system. *JMCP* **2010**, *16*, 185–195. [CrossRef] [PubMed]
8. Smith, M.; Giuliano, M.R.; Starkowski, M.P. In Connecticut: Improving patient medication management in primary care. *Health Aff.* **2011**, *30*, 646–654. [CrossRef] [PubMed]
9. Turner, K.; Buu, J.; Kuzel, M.; Van Wagoner, E.; Berrett, G. Early Implementation of comprehensive medication management within an academic medical center primary care pharmacy team. *Innov. Pharm.* **2020**, *11*, 1. [CrossRef]
10. Livet, M.; Blanchard, C.; Sorensen, T.D.; McClurg, M.R. An Implementation System for Medication Optimization: Operationalizing Comprehensive Medication Management Delivery in Primary Care. *J. Am. Coll. Clin. Pharm.* **2018**, *1*, 14–20. [CrossRef]
11. Pestka, D.L.; Frail, C.K.; Sorge, L.A.; Funk, K.A.; Janke, K.K.; McClurg, M.T.R.; Sorensen, T.D. Development of the comprehensive medication management practice management assessment tool: A resource to assess and prioritize areas for practice improvement. *J. Am. Coll. Clin. Pharm.* **2019**, *3*, 448–454. [CrossRef]
12. Pestka, D.L.; Frail, C.K.; Sorge, L.A.; Funk, K.A.; McClurg, M.T.R.; Sorensen, T.D. The practice management components needed to support comprehensive medication management in primary care clinics. *J. Am. Coll. Clin. Pharm.* **2019**, *3*, 438–447. [CrossRef]

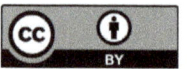

© 2020 by the authors. Licensee MDPI, Basel, Switzerland. This article is an open access article distributed under the terms and conditions of the Creative Commons Attribution (CC BY) license (http://creativecommons.org/licenses/by/4.0/).

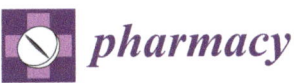 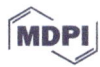

Article

Diabetes-Related Patient Outcomes through Comprehensive Medication Management Delivered by Clinical Pharmacists in a Rural Family Medicine Clinic

Jarred Prudencio * and Michelle Kim

Department of Pharmacy Practice, The Daniel K. Inouye College of Pharmacy, University of Hawaii at Hilo, Hilo, HI 96720, USA; msk@hawaii.edu
* Correspondence: jarredp@hawaii.edu; Tel.:+1-808-932-7703

Received: 1 June 2020; Accepted: 8 July 2020; Published: 9 July 2020

Abstract: Two clinical pharmacy faculty members from a college of pharmacy provide comprehensive medication management in a rural family medicine clinic. The data was assessed for patients with diabetes managed by the pharmacists from 1 January 2017 through to 31 December 2019 to determine the service's impact on patient outcomes. The primary outcome of this study is the change in the goal attainment rates of the three clinical goals of hemoglobin A1c, blood pressure, and appropriate statin therapy after pharmacist intervention. A total of 207 patients were included. At baseline, the patients had an average of 1.13 of the three goals met, improving to an average of 2.02 goals met after pharmacist intervention ($p < 0.001$). At baseline, 4.8% of the patients had met all three clinical goals, improving to 30.9% after pharmacist intervention ($p < 0.001$). There were significant improvements for the individual goal attainment rates of hemoglobin A1c (24.15% vs. 51.21%, $p < 0.001$), blood pressure (42.51% vs. 85.51%, $p < 0.001$), and appropriate statin therapy (45.89% vs. 65.70%, $p < 0.001$). This data adds to the evidence supporting the integration of clinical pharmacists into primary care clinics to improve patient outcomes related to diabetes.

Keywords: diabetes; hypertension; dyslipidemia; primary care; family medicine; comprehensive medication management

1. Introduction

Ambulatory care pharmacy has been a growing area of the clinical pharmacy profession, where pharmacists work with patients in the outpatient setting to ensure safe and effective medication utilization [1]. Although this is becoming a more common area of practice for pharmacists, there has not been a standardization of ambulatory care pharmacy services. The practice models can vary vastly among different clinical sites due to differences in business models, state laws and regulations, and varying degrees of interdisciplinary integration. Ambulatory care pharmacy services can be implemented in a variety of practice settings, including primary care, specialty care, or telehealth clinics. While there is a plethora of evidence that supports ambulatory care pharmacy in each of these settings, the benefit of a clinical pharmacist integrated into a primary care clinic is particularly well documented [2–6]. Although there are varying practices, comprehensive medication management (CMM) is becoming a prominent model for pharmacists embedded in primary care clinics [7]. CMM is a model of service provided by clinical pharmacists that ensures each patient's medication regimen is optimized to ensure the highest safety and efficacy outcomes can be achieved, taking into account patient-specific factors [7].

The Daniel K. Inouye College of Pharmacy (DKICP) at the University of Hawaii at Hilo was established in 2007. The East Hawaii Health Clinic opened in 2009 as a primary care teaching clinic created to educate the future generations of healthcare workers. The clinic includes physicians, nurse practitioners, behavioral health specialists, nurses, and clinical pharmacist faculty members from the DKICP. The learners at this clinic include family medicine physician residents; clinical psychology fellows; and medical, nursing, and pharmacy students. The collaboration between the college and the clinic serves a dual purpose of providing interprofessional patient-centered care and education. As the clinic evolved, so did the clinical pharmacy service. Currently, there are two clinical pharmacist faculty members who have been at this clinic since August 2016 and have established a CMM service. Each pharmacist spends 3 days per week in the clinic and has their own panel of patients to manage, collectively representing 1.2 full-time equivalent (FTE) of pharmacist services. The pharmacists are funded by the DKICP as faculty. The pharmacist faculty precept pharmacy students and educate medical residents on pharmacotherapy topics in the didactic setting and through case consultations.

A common area of focus for pharmacists embedded into primary care clinics is working with patients on the management of diabetes and chronic cardiovascular conditions. Patients with diabetes are at a higher risk of cardiovascular complications, and managing diabetes includes a multitude of factors [8]. Many clinicians focus on three primary goals for patients with diabetes, which are hemoglobin A1c, blood pressure, and cholesterol, otherwise known as "the ABCs of Diabetes" [8]. The American Diabetes Association (ADA) recommends a hemoglobin A1c goal for the average patient with diabetes to be <7%, but a more stringent goal of <6.5% or a less stringent goal of <8% are often considered, depending on patient-specific factors [9]. The blood pressure goal of <140/90 mmHg is also commonly utilized for patients with diabetes [9,10]. While some organizations recommend a blood pressure goal of <130/80 mmHg, the ADA and the Eighth Joint National Committee (JNC8) recommended goal of <140/90 mmHg was chosen for this study [9,10]. Although cholesterol is a concern for patients with diabetes, current clinical practice guidelines focus primarily on utilizing a moderate-to-high intensity statin for patients with diabetes, as opposed to specific lipid panel goals [9,11]. When providing CMM for patients with diabetes, clinicians focus on ensuring that the patient meets these three clinical goals in order to achieve adequate chronic disease state control and prevent future complications. The goal of this study is to assess the impact that a clinical pharmacist-led CMM service has on outcomes for patients with diabetes, as evidenced by changes in the goal attainment rates for hemoglobin A1c, blood pressure, and appropriate statin therapy before and after the pharmacist intervention.

2. Materials and Methods

This study was conducted as a retrospective chart review and was approved by the University of Hawaii Institutional Review Board (Approval Protocol #2018-00938). The electronic medical records (EMR) were reviewed for patients who had at least one appointment with a clinical pharmacist between 1 January 2017 and 31 December 2019.

Patients were scheduled for CMM appointments with the clinical pharmacists through two different avenues. First, the patients could be referred by their primary care provider (PCP). Anecdotally, the majority of patient appointments were scheduled through this route. The majority of referrals from PCPs to the CMM service were due to uncontrolled diabetes, medication nonadherence, or a need for medication education and counseling. Second, patients could be identified by the clinical pharmacists through EMR review due to uncontrolled chronic conditions or potential polypharmacy issues. EMR review was primarily conducted in the first few months of the start of the service, and as the PCPs gained familiarity with the service, the referrals increased over time and less time was spent doing EMR review outreach. In both instances, the patient was then scheduled by the clerical staff and added onto the pharmacist's panel of patients for an in-person visit.

The pharmacist appointments were all 40 min in duration and were conducted as in-person visits to the clinic. While each appointment may not take the full 40 min, this time was set to allow for an in-depth discussion between the pharmacist and the patient regarding their chronic conditions, medications, and lifestyle. This time also allowed for the incorporation of pharmacy student learners to participate in patient appointments. A comprehensive medication reconciliation was completed at the start of each visit to clarify any medication discrepancies or nonadherence. The pharmacist then spends the remainder of the visit providing motivational interviewing, medication, and lifestyle counseling, and clarifying any questions the patient may have. Both pharmacists have a progressive collaborative practice agreement (CPA) with all the physicians in this clinic. The CPA was created by the pharmacist faculty in collaboration with the clinic's medical director. There is no specific credentialing or privileging process included in the CPA, as it is specific to the two DKICP faculty members, who are vetted by the clinic's medical director and administration team during the hiring process. The CPA allows the pharmacist to make changes to the patient's medication regimen including initiating, adjusting, or discontinuing any non-controlled prescription medications. The CPA does not include specific medications, circumstances, or treatment protocols that the pharmacist must follow. Instead, the CPA is openly worded to allow the pharmacist to select drug changes based on their own clinical judgement and knowledge of evidence-based medicine. The CPA also allows the pharmacist to order any relevant laboratory tests that the patient may need and is able to renew prescriptions that are needed. After making the necessary adjustments and providing education to the patient, the patient is then scheduled for a future follow-up appointment with the pharmacist or the PCP based on the discretion of the pharmacist. In both scenarios, the pharmacist is responsible for following up on any results from laboratory tests they order, whether that is discussing results with the patients directly or communicating with the PCP to relay that information. Patients are continuously managed by the pharmacist until their medication regimens remain stable and there is no immediate need for follow-up CMM appointments. At that point, the patients will follow up with their PCP for general wellness appointments and can be rescheduled for a CMM appointment with the pharmacist should the need arise again in the future.

Although the clinical pharmacy service truly is focused on comprehensive medication management as opposed to disease-specific management, the majority of patients referred to the CMM service have been for diabetes management. This is likely due to these pharmacists' specific expertise in diabetes management and because a large portion of diabetes management is based on pharmacotherapy [9]. This clinic is located in a rural city, and patients do not readily have access to endocrinologists or dieticians, which adds to the reasons why the majority of patient referrals are for diabetes. For each of these patients, the 3 primary goals set are attaining a controlled hemoglobin A1c level (patient-specific but typically <7% or <8%), a blood pressure of <140/90 mmHg, and a prescription of a moderate-to-high intensity statin [9–11]. Each goal is set by the clinical pharmacist depending on the specific patient.

To be included in the study analysis, patients must have had a diagnosis of type 1 or type 2 diabetes and have had at least 1 appointment with a pharmacist for CMM. The patients were further excluded from the analysis if they were under 18 years of age or did not have an updated hemoglobin A1c or blood pressure reading after their CMM visit. The primary outcome of this study was the composite of goal attainment rates for patients with diabetes, measured as pre-pharmacist intervention (baseline) and post-pharmacist intervention. The additional secondary outcomes of this study include specific goal attainment rates for hemoglobin A1c, blood pressure, and statin prescription. The blood pressure and hemoglobin A1c values from the initial visit were documented as the baseline value, and the blood pressure and hemoglobin A1c values at the last pharmacist visit were documented as the post-pharmacist intervention value. Other included outcomes are changes in the average hemoglobin A1c and blood pressure, in addition to changes in the number and types of medications used to manage diabetes, hypertension, and dyslipidemia. Statistical analyses were conducted using paired t-tests and McNemar tests and conducted as a per protocol analysis.

3. Results

Over the three-year period, there were a total of 1600 CMM visits with 337 patients managed by the clinical pharmacists between 1 January 2017 and 31 December 2019. Of the 337 patients seen by the CMM service, 224 (66.5%) had a diagnosis of diabetes. These 224 patients had a total of 1417 visits, representing 88.5% of the CMM visits. Of the 224, 17 patients were excluded, leaving a total of 207 patients to be included in the study analysis. Of the 17 excluded patients, 2 patients were under the age of 18 years, and 15 patients did not have an updated hemoglobin A1c after their CMM visit.

Prior to the patients receiving any pharmacy interventions, 10 (4.8%) patients were able to attain all three of the primary clinical goals (a patient-specific controlled hemoglobin A1c level of <7% or <8%, a blood pressure of <140/90 mmHg, and a prescription of a moderate-to-high intensity statin). There were 43 (20.8%) patients that had not met any of the three goals at baseline, and about half (50.7%) of the patients had met one of the three goals. The most common goal attained at baseline was being prescribed an appropriate statin (45.89%). The full baseline characteristics can be found in Table 1.

Table 1. Baseline characteristics (N = 207).

CHARACTERISTIC	PATIENT GROUP (N = 207)
MEAN AGE	56.8 years
FEMALE GENDER, %	49.3
AVERAGE A1C, %	9.42
TYPE 2 DIABETES, N (%)	191 (92.27)
AT A1C GOAL, N (%)	50 (24.15)
AVERAGE SBP	140 mmHg
AVERAGE DBP	79.2 mmHg
AT BLOOD PRESSURE GOAL, N (%)	88 (42.51)
AT STATIN GOAL, N (%)	95 (45.89)
0 OF 3 GOALS MET, N (%)	43 (20.8)
1 OF 3 GOALS MET, N (%)	105 (50.7)
2 OF 3 GOALS MET, N (%)	49 (23.7)
3 OF 3 GOALS MET, N (%)	10 (4.8)

There was a significant increase in the composite of goal attainment rates after the clinical pharmacy interventions, representing the primary objective of the study as depicted in Figure 1 ($p < 0.001$). A total of 64 (30.9%) patients had met all three primary goals after the CMM visits, for an increase of 26.1 percentage points. Overall, 96.1% of all the patients had met at least one of the primary study goals after working with the pharmacist. At baseline, the average amount of goals met was 1.13, and this increased to an average of 2.02 after the CMM ($p < 0.001$).

The secondary objectives of individual goal attainment rates of hemoglobin A1c, hypertension, and appropriate statin prescription were all found to be significantly improved after pharmacy intervention, as depicted in Figure 2. Prior to any pharmacy appointments, 50 (24.15%) patients had a controlled hemoglobin A1c at baseline but after the clinical pharmacy interventions, and 106 patients (51.21%) had reached their A1c goal, for an improvement of 27.06 percentage points ($p < 0.001$). At baseline, 88 (45.21%) patients had a blood pressure considered to be controlled. After the pharmacy interventions, these patients' blood pressure had significantly improved, with 177 (85.51%) of patients reaching their blood pressure goal ($p < 0.001$). A total of 95 (45.89%) patients were prescribed an appropriate statin at baseline, and after pharmacy interventions 136 (65.7%) patients had met their statin goal, for an increase of 19.8 percentage points ($p < 0.001$).

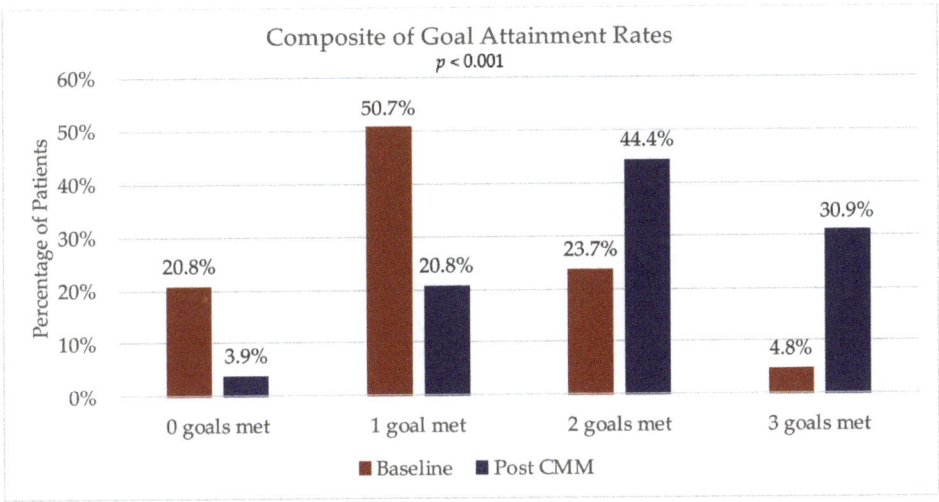

Figure 1. Primary outcome: change in composite of goal attainment rates with comprehensive medication management (CMM).

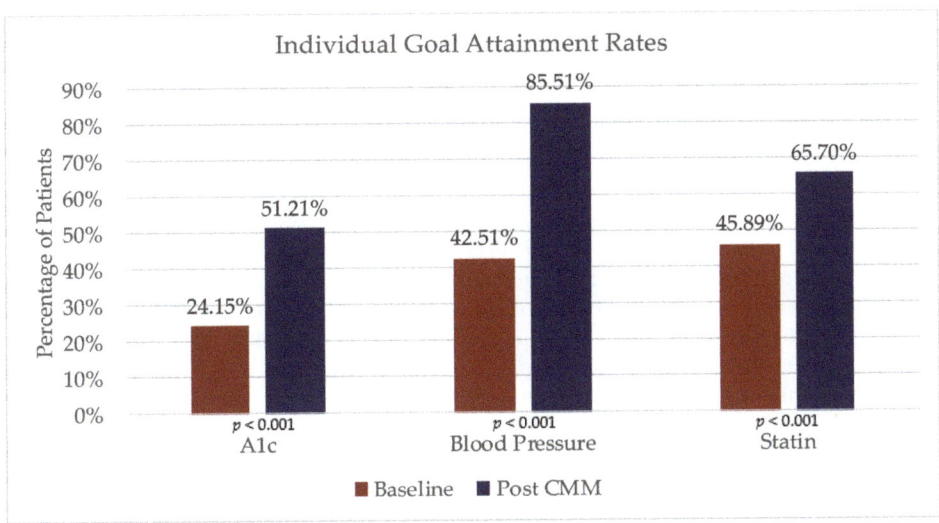

Figure 2. Secondary outcomes: change in individual goal attainment rates with CMM.

The average hemoglobin A1c for all the patients at baseline was 9.4%. After the pharmacy clinical interventions, the hemoglobin A1c had decreased by 1.76 percentage points to an average of 7.66% ($p < 0.001$). When reviewing only patients with uncontrolled diabetes (baseline A1c above goal), the hemoglobin A1c average at baseline was 10.35% and had an even larger decrease of 2.23 percentage points to an average of 8.12%. A full analysis of the changes in hemoglobin A1c can be found in Table 2. The average number of anti-diabetic medications the patients were taking at baseline was 1.66, with the majority already having been prescribed metformin (60.2%). After pharmacy intervention, the average number of diabetes medications had only slightly increased to 1.81. The most common addition to a patient's medication regimen was the increasing use of a GLP-1 agonist. A full breakdown of changes in diabetes medications utilized by drug class can be found in Table 3.

Table 2. Changes in hemoglobin A1c.

	MEAN A1C BASELINE	MEAN A1C POST CMM	MEAN A1C CHANGE	p-Value
ALL PATIENTS (N = 207)	9.42	7.66	−1.76	$p < 0.001$
UNCONTROLLED AT BASELINE (N = 157)	10.35	8.12	−2.23	$p < 0.001$
CONTROLLED AT BASELINE (N = 50)	6.52	6.23	−0.29	$p = 0.001$
TYPE 2 DIABETES (N = 191)	9.27	7.51	−1.77	$p < 0.001$
TYPE 1 DIABETES (N = 16)	11.2	9.54	−1.66	$p < 0.001$
GOAL A1C < 7% (N = 155)	9.4	7.52	−1.88	$p < 0.001$
GOAL A1C < 8% (N = 52)	9.48	8.08	−1.4	$p < 0.001$

Table 3. Changes in anti-diabetic medications for patients with type 2 diabetes (N = 191).

MEDICATION TYPE	BASELINE [N, (%)]	POST CMM [N, (%)]	CHANGE [N, (%)]
METFORMIN	115 (60.2)	116 (60.7)	1 (0.5)
SULFONYLUREAS	34 (17.8)	27 (14.1)	−7 (−3.7)
THIAZOLIDINEDIONES	2 (1)	3 (1.6)	1 (0.5)
SODIUM-GLUCOSE TRANSPORT PROTEIN 2 INHIBITORS	3 (1.6)	11 (5.8)	8 (4.2)
DIPEPTIDYL PEPTIDASE 4 INHIBITORS	13 (6.8)	25 (13.1)	12 (6.3)
GLUCAGON-LIKE PEPTIDE-1 AGONISTS	14 (7.3)	41 (21.5)	27 (14.2)
BASAL INSULIN	90 (47)	91 (47.6)	1 (0.5)
PRANDIAL INSULIN	44 (23)	33 (17.3)	−11 (−5.7)

The average systolic blood pressure (SBP) of patients was reduced from 140 mmHg at baseline to 130.2 mmHg after the CMM visits ($p < 0.001$). A total of 119 patients started off with an uncontrolled blood pressure (BP > 140/90 mmHg), with an average of 152/83 mmHg. After CMM, these patients had a significant improvement in their blood pressure, for a 17 mmHg decrease in SBP and a 6 mmHg decrease in diastolic blood pressure (DBP), for an average blood pressure of 135/77 mmHg. A full description of the blood pressure changes can be found in Table 4. At baseline, the average number of anti-hypertensive medications prescribed per patient was 1.56, and this increased slightly to 1.69 after pharmacy intervention. A description of the changes in antihypertensive medications can be found in Table 5.

Table 4. Changes in blood pressure (BP).

	MEAN BP BASELINE	MEAN BP POST CMM	MEAN CHANGE
ALL PATIENTS (N = 207), SBP	140	130.2	−9.8
ALL PATIENTS (N = 207), DBP	79.2	76	−3.2
UNCONTROLLED AT BASELINE (N = 119), SBP	151.9	134.9	−17
UNCONTROLLED AT BASELINE (N = 119), DBP	83.4	77.2	−6.2
CONTROLLED AT BASELINE (N = 88), SBP	123.9	123.7	−0.2
CONTROLLED AT BASELINE (N = 88), DBP	73.6	74.4	0.8

Table 5. Changes in antihypertension medications (N = 207).

MEDICATION TYPE	BASELINE [N, (%)]	POST CMM [N, (%)]	CHANGE [N, (%)]
ACE INHIBITORS	90 (43.3)	84 (40.6)	−6 (−2.7)
ANGIOTENSIN II RECEPTOR BLOCKERS	47 (22.6)	56 (27.1)	9 (4.5)
THIAZIDE DIURETICS	24 (11.5)	33 (15.9)	9 (4.5)
CALCIUM CHANNEL BLOCKERS	44 (21.1)	52 (25.1)	8 (3.9)
BETA BLOCKERS	79 (38)	85 (41.1)	6 (3.1)
OTHERS	35 (16.8)	32 (15.5)	−3 (−1.3)

Both the ADA and the American College of Cardiology/American Heart Association (ACC/AHA) recommend that all the patients with diabetes between the ages of 40 and 75 years old be prescribed a moderate-to-high intensity statin to decrease the risk of an atherosclerotic cardiovascular disease (ASCVD) event [9,11]. When focusing specifically on the patients between the ages of 40 and 75 years old, about half (51.3%) were on an appropriately dosed statin at baseline. For those between 40 and 75 years old, the results had improved even more, with 72.5% of those patients meeting their statin goal after CMM. In addition to statin therapy, ezetimibe and omega-3 acid ethyl esters were prescribed in a small number of patients. A full list of the changes to lipid-lowering medications can be found in Table 6.

Table 6. Changes in lipid-lowering medications (N = 207).

MEDICATION TYPE	BASELINE [N, (%)]	POST CMM [N, (%)]	CHANGE [N, (%)]
HIGH INTENSITY STATINS	58 (28)	90 (43.5)	32 (15.5)
MODERATE INTENSITY STATINS	38 (18.4)	46 (22.2)	8 (3.8)
LOW INTENSITY STATINS	7 (3.4)	1 (0.5)	−6 (−2.9)
NON-STATINS	8 (3.9)	14 (6.8)	6 (2.9)

4. Discussion

The data analyzed in this study demonstrates that clinical pharmacists can have positive impacts on patients with diabetes in the primary care setting of a rural healthcare clinic. The improvement in the outcomes of goal attainment rates and decreases in hemoglobin A1c and blood pressure are consistent with findings in other studies [2–6]. The improvement in the primary outcome was statistically and clinically significant. As noted in Figure 1, there is a general shift in improvements in goal attainment after the pharmacist-provided CMM visits. While this primary outcome of goal attainment may be viewed as a surrogate marker for disease control, there are data supporting that achieving controlled glycemic and blood pressure levels with an appropriately dosed statin significantly decreases the risk of long-term complications, including microvascular and macrovascular complications [12–14].

The utilization of the progressive collaborative practice agreement is a key element of this CMM service. Without the CPA, the clinical service could not be as efficient, as the pharmacist would need to discuss every recommendation with the physician, which would in turn lead to an increased workload for the physicians. Leveraging this progressive CPA allowed the pharmacists to work at the top of their scope, being readily able to adjust medications based on patient-specific factors.

The data reported in this study represent patient outcomes over three years of this CMM service. While the pharmacists did spend a significant amount of time working with patients to optimize their medication regimens, the patients averaged only 2.23 CMM visits per year. Some patients required only 1 visit per year, while others required up to 11 visits per year. The number of visits needed depended on the severity of the patient's conditions, the types of medications being used, and the amount of patient counseling that was needed to be provided.

Although there was only a minor increase in the number of anti-diabetic and antihypertensive medications prescribed, the hemoglobin A1c and blood pressure control both improved significantly. This improvement could be attributed to the pharmacist making adjustments to the dosing for the current medications the patient was already taking or switching the patient to an alternative medication, as opposed to simply adding on additional medications. For example, there was an increase in the use of GLP-1 agonists and a decrease in the use of sulfonylureas and prandial insulin. This type of change is consistent with the recent changes to the ADA guideline recommendations for using a GLP-1 agonist as a second-line agent after metformin due to the increasing trials showing the benefits of using this medication class in preventing a cardiovascular event [9]. In addition to medication changes, the pharmacist provided extensive medication and lifestyle education and support throughout the process, which could contribute to the improvements in the A1c and blood pressure lowering without a large increase in medication usage.

In addition to the patient outcomes data presented in this article, there have been many anecdotal benefits of having a pharmacist embedded in a primary care clinic. Other providers, such as attending physicians, medical residents, nurse practitioners, and nurses, have frequently expressed that having a clinical pharmacist as part of the interdisciplinary team is invaluable. Although this clinic has not administered a formal provider satisfaction survey regarding pharmacist-led CMM, other studies in the literature have demonstrated that pharmacists in primary care are well-received by other providers [15–18]. One study that surveyed 114 primary care providers reported that PCPs believed that the addition of a clinical pharmacist has a highly positive impact on patient care and would highly recommend that other primary care practices integrate a clinical pharmacist. Additionally, that survey reported that 58.78% of respondents believed diabetes was the most valuable disease-focused pharmacy service, and an additional 9.65% of respondents believed it to be hypertension [15]. While the results from that survey cannot be directly applied to this current study, the CMM model has received great feedback from PCPs that highly value and appreciate the service. In addition to providing CMM, the pharmacists in this clinic are also frequently consulted for drug information questions, medication access concerns, or other informal consults. In fact, the success of this CMM service has led to the planned expansion of CMM services to other primary care clinics within this institution.

A limitation of this research analysis is the lack of a patient control group without a clinical pharmacist. Without this control group, it cannot be directly stated that the clinical pharmacy service can improve these patient outcomes to a higher degree than other types of clinicians. Given that this analysis is of patient data from a small rural health clinic, a control group was not logistically possible. Other patients in the clinic who were not seen by the clinical pharmacy team would not be an appropriate comparison, as the patients seen by the clinical pharmacy team are often more complex compared to those solely managed by the PCP. Additionally, the clinic is an interdisciplinary teaching clinic and the majority of PCPs are family medicine resident physicians. The clinical pharmacists frequently provide undocumented and informal consultations with the physicians, so utilizing other patients in the clinic could not be a definite control group. Without the control group, it can still be inferred that the clinical pharmacy service has had positive impacts on patient outcomes as evidenced by the pre- and post-improvements in chronic disease state outcomes. Other studies have included the use of a control group and have reported improved outcomes in the group that includes a pharmacist [6,19–25]. Although this current study does not include a control group, the improvements in goal attainment and decreases in hemoglobin A1c and blood pressure are consistent with the findings from the other studies. For example, one study conducted at a different institution compared clinics with a pharmacist and clinics without a pharmacist, utilizing the same primary outcome of the composite of goal attainment rates for A1c, blood pressure, and statin therapy. The study concluded that the clinics with the integration of a pharmacist had higher goal attainment rate improvements than the clinics without the pharmacist [6]. Another limitation of this analysis is regarding the dyslipidemia treatment goal. For the purposes of this analysis, the dyslipidemia goal was set as the prescription of a moderate-to-high intensity statin, which is generally recommended for the majority of patients with diabetes aged 40–75 years old. This study did include patients outside of the 40–75 year range and did not assess whether or not a patient had clinical ASCVD or a severely elevated low-density lipoprotein (LDL) at baseline, which are indications for high-intensity statin therapy. The current ACC/AHA guidelines also have added the addition of a secondary LDL goal of <100 mg/dL for patients with diabetes after being prescribed a moderate-to-high intensity or maximally tolerated statin [11]. The LDL levels were not assessed in this data analysis. Additionally, contraindications for statin therapy were not assessed in the data analysis. There may have been reasons why not all the patients were prescribed the statin, including whether they had previously not tolerated a statin medication, had a history of rhabdomyolysis, or had liver dysfunction.

Future areas of interest in this research topic include developing additional methods to analyze a CMM service. Given that pharmacy services in primary care clinics can have widely varying models from different institutions, no formal CMM metric or analysis has become the gold standard. Areas of consideration for future research include CMM effects on patient hospitalization rates, medication adverse effect rates, and quality of life. The outcomes reported in this analysis are focused primarily on the patient outcomes related to diabetes. While this does provide results for the majority of patients managed by this service (61.4% of the total CMM patients were included in this analysis), there were a significant number of patients that did not have diabetes and were managed by the clinical pharmacy service. These patients could have been referred to the pharmacy service for polypharmacy concerns or the management of other non-diabetes chronic conditions such as COPD, heart failure, or anticoagulation management. Given that CMM services provide management for a large range of conditions, it is difficult to determine a single primary outcome to research to assess the entire service.

This clinical pharmacy service additionally has plans to expand in the future. Currently, the authors are in the process of adding an additional clinical pharmacist to provide a similar CMM service at the other primary care clinics within the network of this institution. This expansion was requested by the medical director who has seen first-hand the added value and improved patient care by integrating a pharmacist. In addition to expanding this model to the other clinics, the authors are considering expanding the service to include a transition of care service. The clinic is located on the same campus as a hospital, where PCPs have inpatient privileges and rotate through the inpatient wards to manage their patients when admitted. This provides a great set-up to have a transition of care service, which would include a patient handoff from acute care clinical pharmacists to the ambulatory care clinical pharmacists for post-discharge management.

5. Conclusions

This study has shown that having a clinical pharmacist integrated in a primary care setting has significantly benefited patients with type 1 and type 2 diabetes in obtaining improved control of their condition. The pharmacist's expertise in CMM management positively impacts patient care, and an expansion of CMM services should be considered.

Author Contributions: Conceptualization, J.P. and M.K.; Data curation, J.P. and M.K.; Formal analysis, J.P. and M.K.; Investigation, J.P. and M.K.; Methodology, J.P. and M.K.; Project administration, J.P.; Writing—original draft, J.P. and M.K.; Writing—review & editing, J.P. and M.K. All authors have read and agreed to the published version of the manuscript.

Funding: This research received no external funding.

Acknowledgments: The authors would like to acknowledge the fellow healthcare providers at the East Hawaii Health Clinic—1190 Primary Care—for their contribution to the interprofessional healthcare analyzed in this study.

Conflicts of Interest: The authors declare no conflict of interest.

References

1. Ambulatory Care Pharmacy, Board of Pharmacy Specialties. Available online: https://www.bpsweb.org/media/ambulatory-care-pharmacy-fact-sheet/ (accessed on 1 April 2020).
2. Chisholm-Burns, M.A.; Lee, J.K.; Spivey, C.A.; Slack, M.; Herrier, R.N.; Hall-Lipsy, E.; Zivin, J.G.; Abraham, I.; Palmer, J.; Martin, J.R.; et al. U.S. pharmacists' effect as team members on patient care: Systematic review and meta-analysis. *Med. Care* **2010**, *48*, 923–933. [CrossRef]
3. Tan, E.C.K.; Stewart, K.; Elliott, R.A.; George, J. Pharmacist services provided in general practice clinics: A systematic review and meta-analysis. *Res. Soc. Adm. Pharm.* **2014**, *10*, 608–622. [CrossRef] [PubMed]
4. Ip, E.J.; Shah, B.M.; Yu, J.; Chan, J.; Nguyen, L.T.; Bhatt, D.C. Enhancing diabetes care by adding a pharmacist to the primary care team. *Am. J. Health Syst. Pharm.* **2013**, *70*, 877–886. [CrossRef] [PubMed]
5. Jacobs, M.; Sherry, P.S.; Taylor, L.M.; Amato, M.; Tataronis, G.R.; Cushing, G. Pharmacist Assisted Medication Program Enhancing the Regulation of Diabetes (PAMPERED) study. *J. Am. Pharm. Assoc.* **2012**, *52*, 613–621. [CrossRef] [PubMed]
6. Prudencio, J.; Cutler, T.; Roberts, S.; Marin, S.; Wilson, M. The Effect of Clinical Pharmacist-Led Comprehensive Medication Management on Chronic Disease State Goal Attainment in a Patient-Centered Medical Home. *J. Manag. Care Spec. Pharm.* **2018**, *24*, 423–429. [CrossRef] [PubMed]
7. American College of Clinical Pharmacy (ACCP). Standards of practice for clinical pharmacists. *Pharmacotherapy* **2014**, *34*, 794–797. [CrossRef] [PubMed]
8. ABCs of Diabetes, Diabetes Self Management. Available online: https://www.diabetesselfmanagement.com/managing-diabetes/complications-prevention/taking-diabetes-to-heart/abcs-of-diabetes/ (accessed on 3 March 2020).
9. American Diabetes Association. Standards of medical care in diabetes—2020. *Diabetes Care* **2020**, *43*, S1–S212. [CrossRef]
10. James, P.A.; Oparil, S.; Carter, B.L.; Cushman, W.C.; Dennison-Himmelfarb, C.; Handler, J.; Lackland, D.T.; LeFevre, M.L.; MacKenzie, T.D.; Ogedegbe, O.; et al. 2014 Evidence-based guideline for the management of high blood pressure in adults: Report from the panel members appointed to the eigth joint national committee (JNC 8). *JAMA* **2014**, *311*, 507–520. [CrossRef]
11. Grundy, S.M.; Stone, N.J.; Bailey, A.L.; Beam, C.; Birtcher, K.K.; Blumenthal, R.S.; Braun, L.T.; de Ferranti, S.; Faiella-Tommasino, J.; Forman, D.E.; et al. 2018 AHA/ACC/AACVPR/AAPA/ABC/ACPM/ADA/AGS/APhA/ASPC/NLA/PCNA guideline on the management of blood cholesterol: A report of the american college of cardiology/american heart association task force on clinical practice guidelines. *Circulation* **2019**, *139*, e1082–e1143.
12. Wieczorek, A.; Rys, P.; Skrzekowska-Baran, I.; Malecki, M. The role of surrogate endpoints in the evaluation of efficacy and safety of therapeutic interventions in diabetes mellitus. *Rev. Diabet. Stud.* **2008**, *5*, 128–135. [CrossRef]
13. Colhoun, H.M.; Betteridge, D.J.; Durrington, P.N.; Hitman, G.A.; Neil, H.A.; Livingstone, S.J.; Thomason, M.J.; Mackness, M.I.; Charlton-Menys, V.; Fuller, J.H.; Cards Investigators. Primary prevention of cardiovascular disease with atorvastatin in type 2 diabetes in the collaborative atorvastatin diabetes Study (CARDS): Multicentre randomised placebo-controlled trial. *Lancet* **2004**, *364*, 685–696. [CrossRef]
14. Emdin, C.A.; Rahimi, K.; Neal, B.; Callender, T.; Perkovic, V.; Patel, A. Blood pressure lowering in type 2 diabetes: A systematic review and meta-analysis. *JAMA* **2015**, *313*, 603–615. [CrossRef] [PubMed]
15. Truong, H.; Kroehl, M.E.; Lewis, C.; Pettigrew, R.; Bennett, M.; Saseen, J.J.; Trinkley, K.E. Clinical pharmacists in primary care: Provider satisfaction and perceived impact on quality of care provided. *SAGE Open Med.* **2017**, *5*, 2050312117713911. [CrossRef] [PubMed]
16. Al-Omar, L.T.; Anderson, S.L.; Cizmic, A.D.; Vlasimsky, T.B. Implementation of a pharmacist-led diabetes management protocol. *Am. Health Drug Benefits* **2019**, *12*, 14–20.
17. Wilson, C.G.; Park, I.; Sutherland, S.E.; Ray, L. Assessing pharmacist-led annual wellness visits: Interventions made and patient and physician satisfaction. *J. Am. Pharm. Assoc.* **2015**, *55*, 449–454. [CrossRef] [PubMed]
18. Collins, C.; Kramer, A.; O'Day, M.E.; Low, M.B. Evaluation of patient and provider satisfaction with a pharmacist-managed lipid clinic in a Veterans affairs medical center. *Am. J. Health Syst. Pharm.* **2006**, *63*, 1723–1727. [CrossRef] [PubMed]

19. Narain, K.D.; Doppee, D.; Li, N.; Moreno, G.; Bell, D.S.; Do, A.L.; Follett, R.W.; Mangione, C.M. An effectiveness evaluation of a primary care-embedded clinical pharmacist-led intervention among blacks with diabetes. *J. Gen. Intern Med.* **2020**, 1–7. [CrossRef] [PubMed]
20. Abdulrhim, S.; Sankaralingam, S.; Ibrahim, M.I.; Awaisu, A. The impact of pharmacist care on diabetes outcomes in primary care settings: An umbrella review of published systematic reviews. *Prim. Care Diabetes* **2020**. [CrossRef]
21. Fink, R.M.; Mooney, E.M.; Saseen, J.J.; Billups, S.J. A comparison of clinical pharmacist management of type 2 diabetes versus usual care in a federally qualified health center. *Pharm. Pract.* **2019**, *17*, 1618. [CrossRef]
22. Huff, J.M.; Falter, R.A.; Scheinberg, N. Retrospective comparison of appropriate statin use between patients with diabetes in the primary care setting managed by pharmacists or internal medicine providers. *Diabetes Spectr.* **2019**, *32*, 349–354. [CrossRef]
23. Schultz, J.L.; Horner, K.E.; McDanel, D.L.; Miller, M.L.; Beranek, R.L.; Jacobsen, R.B.; Sly, N.J.; Miller, A.C.; Mascardo, L.A. Comparing clinical outcomes of a pharmacist-managed diabetes clinic to usual physician-based care. *J. Pharm. Pract.* **2018**, *31*, 268–271. [CrossRef] [PubMed]
24. Benedict, A.W.; Spence, M.M.; Sie, J.L.; Chin, H.A.; Ngo, C.D.; Salmingo, J.F.; Vidaurreta, A.T.; Rashid, N. Evaluation of a pharmacist-managed diabetes program in a primary care setting within an integrated health care system. *J. Manag. Care Spec. Pharm.* **2018**, *24*, 114–122. [CrossRef] [PubMed]
25. Siaw, M.Y.; Ko, Y.; Malone, D.C.; Tsou, K.Y.; Lew, Y.J.; Foo, D.; Tan, E.; Chan, S.C.; Chia, A.; Sinaram, S.S.; et al. Impact of pharmacist-involved collaborative care on the clinical, humanistic, and cost outcomes of high-risk patients with type 2 diabetes (IMPACT): A randomized controlled trial. *J. Clin. Pharm. Ther.* **2017**, *42*, 475–482. [CrossRef] [PubMed]

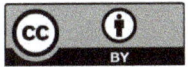

© 2020 by the authors. Licensee MDPI, Basel, Switzerland. This article is an open access article distributed under the terms and conditions of the Creative Commons Attribution (CC BY) license (http://creativecommons.org/licenses/by/4.0/).

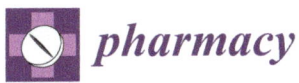

Article

Practice Transformation Driven through Academic Partnerships

Renee Robinson [1,*], Cara Liday [2], Anushka Burde [2], Tracy Pettinger [2], Amy Paul [1], Elaine Nguyen [3], John Holmes [2], Megan Penner [1], Angela Jaglowicz [1], Nathan Spann [3], Julia Boyle [3], Michael Biddle [3], Brooke Buffat [2], Kevin Cleveland [3], Brecon Powell [2] and Christopher Owens [2]

1. Department of Pharmacy Practice and Administrative Sciences, College of Pharmacy, Idaho State University, Anchorage Campus, Anchorage, AK 99508, USA; paulamy@isu.edu (A.P.); pennmeg2@isu.edu (M.P.); jaglange@isu.edu (A.J.)
2. Department of Pharmacy Practice and Administrative Sciences, College of Pharmacy, Idaho State University, Pocatello Campus, Pocatello, ID 83209, USA; lidacara@isu.edu (C.L.); burdanu1@isu.edu (A.B.); petttra1@isu.edu (T.P.); holmjohn@isu.edu (J.H.); bbuffat@isu.edu (B.B.); powebrec@isu.edu (B.P.); owenchri@isu.edu (C.O.)
3. Department of Pharmacy Practice and Administrative Sciences, College of Pharmacy, Idaho State University, Meridian Campus, Meridian, ID 83642, USA; nguyelai@isu.edu (E.N.); spannath@isu.edu (N.S.); boyljuli@isu.edu (J.B.); biddmich@isu.edu (M.B.); clevkevi@isu.edu (K.C.)
* Correspondence: robiren2@isu.edu; Tel.: +1-907-786-6233

Received: 30 May 2020; Accepted: 7 July 2020; Published: 14 July 2020

Abstract: Evidence-based interventions have been shown to improve the quality of patient care, reduce costs, and improve overall health outcomes; however, adopting new published research and knowledge into practice has historically been slow, and requires an active, systematic approach to engage clinicians and healthcare administrators in the required change. Pharmacists have been identified as important agents of change and can enhance care delivery in primary care settings through evidence-based interventions. Utilizing the Consolidated Framework for Implementation Research (CFIR) we identify, assess, and share barriers and facilitators to program development, as well as growth and expansion efforts across five discrete, university-subsidized, embedded-pharmacy practices in primary care. We identified two overarching modifiable factors that influence current and future practice delivery and highlight the role of academia as an incubator for practice change and implementation: Data collection and information sharing. Conceptual frameworks such as CFIR help establish a common vernacular that can be used to facilitate systematic practice site implementation and dissemination of information required to support practice transformation.

Keywords: primary health care; pharmacy; evidence-based pharmacy practice; health outcomes; academic; dissemination; practice transformation; implementation science; quality improvement

1. Introduction

Evidence-based interventions have been shown to improve the quality of care, reduce costs, and improve health and humanistic outcomes [1,2]. However, adopting new published research and knowledge into practice has historically been slow [3,4]. To increase the type and amount of practice-based evidence to drive innovation and subsequently evidence-based practice in all patient care settings, a better support for systematic engagement is needed. Academic pharmacists in clinical teaching and patient care roles are ideally situated to identify and address barriers to implementation, information dissemination, and to establish mechanisms to support lasting practice change.

Pharmacists holding faculty positions (i.e., academic pharmacists) who are embedded in clinical settings have the responsibility of providing direct patient care in collaboration with interprofessional teams as well as facilitating clinical learning experiences for pharmacy students and residents [5]. Such positions may be in healthcare systems, hospitals, primary care clinics, community pharmacies, or other practice settings. In addition to patient care activities and teaching, academic pharmacists often have scholarship responsibilities and are expected to disseminate the results of innovative practice activities. The American Medical Association (AMA) has called for embedding pharmacists into practice as a means of enhancing patient care, raising physician satisfaction, and supporting practice sustainability [6]. In these settings, pharmacists are already driving change in implementation science.

Dissemination and implementation (DI) science is a relatively new discipline that provides a framework for stakeholders (i.e., researchers, clinicians, and healthcare administrators) to identify, interpret, evaluate, and disseminate evidence-based research findings into practice (implementation) [3]. DI intends to bridge the gap between research and practice, translating evidence-based practice and research into real-world settings using conceptual frameworks and translating lessons learned into strategies that fit the daily workflow of a variety of clinical settings. Conceptual frameworks such as those used in DI increase generalizability and interpretability of results, and expedite the application of findings into practice by highlighting factors known to influence the outcomes of interest in this case, implementation of interventions to improve health care delivery by better utilization of pharmacists in the primary care setting.

DI has been used by pharmacists to study practice advancement and implementation in a variety of settings (e.g., community pharmacies in Spain, hospital pharmacies in the US and United Kingdom) [7–9]. However, to our knowledge it has not been used to explore the barriers and facilitators of change pharmacists face when embedded in primary care settings and specifically the role academic pharmacists can play in this incubator of change. There are many DI tools, frameworks, and logic models (project roadmaps) available to assist stakeholders and guide systematic evaluation. The Consolidated Framework for Implementation Research (CFIR) is a construct widely used in health services and pharmacy research for over 20 years [10]. CFIR is intended to be flexible, enabling researchers to tailor the framework to the specific intervention design, factors, and context studied.

In this article, we utilized CFIR and examples from five university-subsidized academic pharmacists to identify and assess barriers and facilitators to the initiation and expansion of embedded-pharmacy practice in primary care. The analysis focused on sharing the embedded pharmacist's experiences with practice implementation, steps taken, and examples of how these changes impacted healthcare delivery and practice at their site (e.g., enhanced medication adherence, reduced adverse events, and improved patient satisfaction). We hope through shared experience in a structured format (CFIR) to guide pharmacists in the US and other countries to support program development and expansion of pharmacist non-dispensing services in primary care.

2. Materials and Methods

To present our approach, we utilize a case series format, informed by a formative cross-site, qualitative investigation of five sites in which the pharmacist was embedded in a primary care setting. All sites were supported by one university system, Idaho State University. Partner healthcare facilities varied in size, organization type (non-profit, for-profit), population served, and geographic location. The practice transformation initiative spanned two rural and frontier states that historically have limited healthcare resources (Idaho and Alaska).

To understand how practice sites experienced and/or were experiencing implementation changes we developed a semi-structured interview guide, scheduled and interviewed pharmacists within the embedded practice site(s). The interview guide focused on the factors surrounding practice transformation and asked embedded pharmacists at the five sites to: (1) Describe the changes made by primary care practice sites to embed the pharmacist faculty within the practice, (2) identify barriers and facilitators to implementation, and (3) share personal experiences of how the embedded pharmacist has engaged in the primary care practice. Questions focused on: (1) How the embedded pharmacist was operationalized in the primary care setting including exploration and installation steps, (2) how the existing practice and workflow functions did or did not support the embedded pharmacist, (3) what was helpful or not helpful during the implementation process, and (4) the pharmacists' perception of how other stakeholders (patients, providers, and the healthcare systems) viewed their addition to the healthcare team. A template analysis approach was used to code interviews with individual embedded pharmacists. As part of the process, codes were refined, coding definitions established, coding rules developed, and interviews coded. CFIR domains and constructs were used to contextualize findings that represented the factors influencing embedded pharmacists' implementation in primary care (Figure 1) [11]. Coded reports were then used to identify whether the finding (and matched construct) exerted a negative, positive, or neutral influence on implementation.

The CFIR is composed of five major domains, each of which may affect an intervention's implementation:	
Intervention characteristics	•Intervention characteristics are features of an intervention that might influence implementation •Eight constructs are included in intervention characteristics (e.g., stakeholders' perceptions about the relative advantage of implementing the intervention, complexity)
Inner setting	•The inner setting is features of the implementing organization that might influence implementation •Twelve constructs are included in inner setting (e.g., implementation climate, leadership engagement)
Outer setting	•The outer setting is features of the external context or environment that might influence implementation •Four constructs are included in outer setting (e.g., external policy and incentives)
Characteristics of individuals	•Characteristics of individuals are those that might influence implementation •Five constructs are included in characteristics of individuals (e.g., knowledge and beliefs about the intervention)
Implementation process	•Implementation process is the strategies or tactics that might influence implementation •Eight constructs are included in to implementation process (e.g., engaging appropriate individuals in the implementation and use of the intervention, reflecting, and evaluating)

Figure 1. Consolidated Framework for Implementation Research (CFIR) domains.

A narrative report of barriers and facilitators identified by site was developed by the desired patient outcome (e.g., improved clinical outcomes, increased medication adherence, and reduced adverse drug events) and was linked to the Centers for Medicare and Medicaid Services (CMS) established core primary care (CPC) functions. CPC functions include insights on practice readiness, care delivery and redesign, actionable performance-based incentives, necessary health information technology (HIT), and data sharing. The five core CPC functions are: (1) Risk-stratified care management, (2) access and continuity, (3) planned care for chronic conditions and preventive care, (4) patient and caregiver engagement, and (5) coordination of care across the medical neighborhood. Similarities, differences, and trends in how the practice sites experienced change were reviewed and summarized. Drawing on the analytic matrices for each program component and CFIR domain, summary tables were developed to visualize barriers and facilitators and support identification of key areas where additional support would be necessary for long-term sustainability.

3. Results

What happened during the embedded pharmacists' implementation? How did various constructs influence operationalization of primary care workflows? What was the impact of the embedded pharmacist on patient clinical outcomes, medication adherence, adverse drug events, and patient satisfaction? The important contextual factors and examples as they relate to practice site implementation, operationalization, and outcomes experienced at the five practice sites are shared below. In Table 1, select factors contributing to perceived readiness (established from interview data) were organized by CFIR domains and CPC components. In Table 2, barriers and facilitators to implementation are presented.

Table 1. Select insights on practice readiness: Relationship between CFIR domains, Centers for Medicare and Medicaid Services (CMS) core primary care functions, and embedded pharmacist experiences and perceptions.

CFIR Domain	CPC Components	Embedded Pharmacist Experiences: Practice Site Findings	Embedded Pharmacist Perceptions: Contributing Factors to Readiness
Intervention characteristics	Care Management Processes - Patient outcomes	Practices faced challenges documenting, coding, and billing for services within established EHR systems.	University subsidized pharmacist and student time served as an incubator for trialing processes, expansion of programs, and establishment of evaluation metrics.
	Access and Continuity - Patient outcomes - Medication adherence	Access to educational, training, and grant resources improved incorporation of evidence-based practice in rural communities and improved access to necessary clinical and payment support resources.	University and grant subsidized pharmacist and student time served as an incubator for development and trialing and expanding of clinical pharmacists' programs for underserved and under-resources communities (e.g., rural residents).
	Planned Chronic and Preventative Care - Adverse drug events - Patient outcomes	Access to educational and training resources improved incorporation of evidence-based practice in rural communities. Better understanding of necessary coding and billing processes were required to provide care and sustain embedded pharmacist service delivery.	University subsidized pharmacist and student time as well as available education and training resources supported embedded pharmacist program management, complex regimen management, and service expansion.
	Patient Engagement - Medication adherence - Patient outcomes	Practice members perceived engagement with patients as vital to improve patient outcomes, self-management, and treatment adherence.	University subsidized pharmacist and student time resulted in increased patient engagement and supported chronic disease self-management.
	Care Coordination - Medication adherence - Patient outcomes - Adverse drug events	Perceived coordination within the patient centered medical home (PCMH) ensured patient follow-up, improved adherence, reduced adverse events, and supported improved patient outcomes.	University subsidized pharmacist and student time reduced clinician burden, improved clinical problem identification, and supported optimization of therapy.
	Care Management Processes - Adverse drug events - Medication adherence - Patient outcomes	Effectively and efficiently addressing patient needs was a common challenge, this included personnel time and economic resources.	Time and resources required to meet patient needs were addressed by embedded pharmacists and students in the primary care clinic. Connecting individuals with medication assistance programs and grant supports.
Outer setting	Access and Continuity	Site health information technology systems and billing infrastructure were unable to support state documentation, coding, and billing requirements required for service provision and sustainability.	Sharing of technology resources, EHR templates, CPAs, policies, and training materials across sites.
	Patient Engagement - Patient outcomes - Medication adherence	Help patients in rural and underserved communities manage chronic health conditions and access necessary supports.	Using the PCMH model, patients in rural and underserved communities received more attention from the healthcare system.
Inner setting	Care Management Processes - Adverse drug events - Patient outcomes	Health information technology systems and billing infrastructure were unable to support documentation, coding, and billing requirements to support service provision, expansion of services, and/or sustainability.	University subsidized pharmacist and grant funding to support training, infrastructure development, advocacy, and improve EHR and billing infrastructure.
	Access and Continuity - Patient outcomes	Embedded pharmacists and students often functioned on a consultant basis and were not present within the primary care clinic due to teaching requirements, resulting in limited access, missed interventions, and sporadic engagement with the team.	Practices with embedded pharmacists' offices centrally located were more accessible to providers and patients and utilized more by the PCMH team.

Table 1. *Cont.*

CFIR Domain	CPC Components	Embedded Pharmacist Experiences: Practice Site Findings	Embedded Pharmacist Perceptions: Contributing Factors to Readiness
	Care Management Processes - Adverse drug events - Patient outcomes - Medication adherence	Primary care provider groups who worked with embedded pharmacists in the past were more likely to work with pharmacists and students to improve/optimize drug therapy.	Primary care practices that worked with embedded pharmacists to establish and modify workflows were more likely to successfully impact patient outcomes, improve medication adherence, identify and reduce adverse drug events.
Characteristics of individuals	Access and Continuity - Adverse drug events - Patient outcomes	Practices that believed in the value of embedded pharmacists worked with healthcare systems to incorporate them into the PCMH and daily practice.	Practices tended to utilize embedded pharmacists and students that were physically available, that rounded with the team, and that participated in clinical activities (e.g., lunch and learns, grand rounds).
	Patient Engagement - Patient outcomes	Patients and staff tend to reach out to individuals with similar values and beliefs.	Healthcare administrators and university providers supported students and pharmacists with whom they have relationships, shared mission, vision, and clinical practice goals.
Implementation process	Care Management Processes - Adverse drug events - Patient outcomes	Shared goals, consistent vernacular and tailored training and supports were required for sustainable practice site improvements.	Co-development of policies, procedures, and workflows is required. Consistent and comprehensive informal and formal training with opportunities for hands-on practice is required for program implementation and sustainability.
	Patient Engagement	Engagement of patients, staff, and providers were required to sustain practice-level improvements.	Healthcare administrators and university providers supported students and pharmacists that add value to the organizations. This is further strengthened when the service is valued by external partners (e.g., insurers).

Table 2. Identified facilitators and barriers to implementation across sites.

Characteristics of Intervention [a]	Inner Setting	Outer Setting	Individuals Involved	Implementation Process
IMPLEMENTATION (Embedded Pharmacist Position, Family Practice Clinic)				
- Subsidized position (university sponsored) - Academic incubator - Connection with educational and training resources - Program expansion	- Physician-owned clinic - Office on site - For profit - Teaching facility for Rx students - Barriers to provider understanding	- Community support - Incentives for students - Unmet patient needs - Provider time constraints	- Pharmacist(s) at site - Intern/Students - Patients (self-efficacy) - Providers (diverse) - University system (Rx)	- Workflow development (enrollment, tracking, delivery) - Engaging with community - Engaging with providers - Educating providers and staff
IMPLEMENTATION (Embedded Pharmacist Position, Internal Medicine Clinic)				
- Subsidized (university sponsored) - Academic incubator - Connection with educational and training resources - Program expansion - Management services offered: Diabetes, hypertension, comprehensive medication reviews	- Primary care clinic - Office on site - Teaching facility for Rx students	- Community support - Incentives for students - Unmet patient needs - Provider time constraints - Larger organization, additional authorization (change slow)	- Pharmacist at site - Intern/Students - Patients (self-efficacy) - Providers (diverse) - University system (Rx) - Healthcare administration - Information technology (IT) - Billing/Finance	- Workflow development (enrollment, tracking, delivery) - Engaging with community - Engaging with providers - Educating providers and staff - Readiness for implementation (IT billing, and finance lagged behind)
IMPLEMENTATION (Embedded Pharmacist Position, Rural Health)				
- Subsidized (university sponsored) - Academic incubator - Connection with educational and training resources - Growing complexity and program expansion	- Primary care clinic (MD owned until 2016) - Office on site - Teaching facility for Rx students	- Community support - Incentives for students - Unmet patient needs - Provider time constraints	- Pharmacist at site - Intern/Students - Patients (self-efficacy) - Providers (diverse) - University system	- Workflow (consultant role) - Engaging with community - Engaging with providers - Educating providers and staff (formal and informal)
IMPLEMENTATION (HIV/AIDs Incubator Project at Community Pharmacy)				
- Subsidized (university sponsored) - Academic incubator - Connection with educational and training resources - Grant funded project (metrics mandated)	- Federally qualified health center (FQHC) - Community Pharmacy - Office on site - Teaching facility for Rx students	- Community support - Unmet patient needs - Provider time constraints - External incentives to participate	- Pharmacist(s) at site - Intern/Students - Patients (incentivized, high resource needs) - University system	- Workflow development (enrollment, tracking, delivery) - Engaging with HIV/AIDs community - Training of staff and patients
IMPLEMENTATION (Embedded Pharmacist Position with Private Medical Group)				
- Subsidized (university sponsored) - Academic incubator for billing - Connection with educational and training resources - Management services offered: Chronic disease management - Healthcare initiated and supported	- Primary care clinic - Office on site - Teaching facility for Rx students	- Community support - Incentives for students - Unmet patient needs - Provider time constraints - External billing	- Pharmacist(s) at site - Intern/Students - Providers (diverse) - University system - Healthcare administration - Information technology (IT) - Billing/Finance	- Workflow development (enrollment, tracking, delivery) - Educating providers and staff - Readiness for implementation (IT, billing and finance lagged behind) - Educating legal (fear of fraud)

[a] Intervention refers to the addition of the embedded pharmacists within the primary care clinic setting.

Clinical outcomes: In 1998, a university-sponsored embedded pharmacist position was established at a for-profit, family practice clinic. This non-dispensing clinical pharmacy position, one of the first of its kind in Idaho, was created as a rotation site for students to complete required advanced pharmacy practice experiences (APPE) in primary care and was fully subsidized by the university.

Initially foreign to patients, providers, and healthcare administrators, it took approximately six years to garner the necessary trust of healthcare providers and administrators for the pharmacist to begin taking on specific tasks/roles to support the clinic providers (e.g., conducting chart reviews, managing anticoagulation therapy). Relationships between the embedded pharmacist and clinic developed over a six-year period starting with collaborating with providers to suggest evidence-based pharmacotherapy recommendations to better meet clinic patient needs. Later, case examples and individual-level health outcome data resulting directly from the embedded pharmacist contributions were shared with providers and healthcare administrators. Improvements in traditional documented health outcomes such as hemoglobin A1c and satisfaction metrics were shared with providers and healthcare teams to demonstrate impact. It is noteworthy that, it was not until the embedded pharmacist became a Certified Diabetes Educator (CDE) that healthcare providers and administrators within the system more fully understood her role as a billable healthcare service provider supporting the combined clinic visit structure. Initially, the primary care practice only supported using billing codes such as 99211 typically used for the evaluation and management of an established patient with minimal presenting problem(s) addressed in approximately 5 min, underbilling for pharmacist time, and health services provided. Over the next 10 years, formal reimbursement and collaborative practice agreements were established with the healthcare facility to enable the embedded pharmacist to independently bill for the non-dispensing services provided and for the pharmacist outcome metrics to be reported with system health metrics to insurers.

In 2007, the university approached a physician-owned clinic to establish another university-subsidized, embedded-pharmacist position within primary care. The physician-owned clinic, located in southeastern Idaho, provided care to rural communities and offered a unique opportunity for the academic pharmacists, along with pharmacy residents and students to identify and address rural health concerns of rural patients. Some clinical providers in this clinic were previously exposed to pharmacy residents and clinical pharmacy services, but were not familiar with all of the available supports an embedded pharmacist could provide within a primary care clinic. It was based on this experience that an embedded position was created.

Over the following 13 years, the scope of pharmacy practice expanded to include management of all health conditions covered within the clinic, focusing on the appropriateness of treatment and monitoring of drug therapy. Acting as part of the team, individual-level metrics were not collected, only team metrics, which demonstrates the level of the clinic commitment to engaging all providers.

Medication adherence: Adherence to prescribed antiretroviral therapy is essential for maintaining viral suppression in patients with human immunodeficiency virus (HIV) and/or acquired immunodeficiency syndrome (AIDS). Poor adherence is associated with an increased risk of drug resistance, opportunistic infection, virologic failure, hospitalizations, and increased mortality [12–16]. Barriers to medication adherence typically revolve around unmet education and fiscal needs, both of which were identified and addressed through increased, focused provider communication facilitated by embedded pharmacists.

In 2014, a University-sponsored non-profit community pharmacy, was awarded a Ryan White Capacity Grant to create and implement a Patient Centered Pharmacy Program (PCPP) in partnership with a Federally Qualified Health Center (FQHC) to improve HIV management and reduce HIV-related health disparities in rural Idaho. Enrollment, tracking, and delivery forms were created, training materials for staff and patients developed, and unique payment support models (e.g., 340B pricing, enrollment in Idaho's AIDS Drug Assistance Program, manufacturer coupon cards, and Ryan White Grant) secured by a pharmacy faculty member over a four-month period. Pharmacy students were likewise employed to support training needs, pair individuals with appropriate payers, and foster an environment conducive to support medication adherence that would not have been possible without university and grant subsidization.

Adverse Drug Events: According to the World Health Organization, an adverse drug reaction (ADR) is a "response to a medication that is noxious and unintended" [17]. Many ADRs are preventable, including known side-effects related to medication administration or a drug-drug interaction, but they may be unexpected, such as an allergic reaction. Approximately 3.5% of all hospital admissions are attributed to an ADR, and as the number and complexity of drug therapies increase, the number of ADRs is expected to rise [18–22].

In the current practice environment, primary care providers face increasing demands on their time (e.g., service and authorization requests, documentation demands) and shorter patient visits, resulting in fewer healthcare issues addressed and diminished patient understanding [23–26]. Time spent on patient education, medication/therapy management, and care coordination is significantly reduced. This reduced time results in a knowledge gap, the "why behind treatment" is unclear and the adverse drug event risk increased, especially in older adults with co-morbid conditions with complex medication regimens [27,28].

In July 2007, an embedded, university-sponsored pharmacist position was established within one of the internal medicine clinics, a clinic responsible for the management of ~1200 mostly older patients per year. The pharmacist works under a Collaborative Practice Agreement (CPA) signed by all the providers (nurse practitioners, physician assistants, and physicians) in the clinic. Patients are referred to the embedded pharmacist for comprehensive medication reviews and chronic disease management of diabetes, hypertension, hyperlipidemia, hyperthyroidism, asthma, and/or chronic obstructive pulmonary disease. A team-based approach to care allows for real-time problem-solving, with healthcare teams working together to make both individual level and program-based care decisions to optimize drug therapy and to prevent ADRs. These co-developed plans decrease inappropriate service utilization, free up providers to focus on their discipline specific scope of practice, and improve health outcomes.

Medication-focused disease management activities that improve adherence and outcomes include medication reconciliation, pre-emptive prior authorization requests, medication substitutions, and ongoing, chronic disease management. Students completing rotations assist with medication reconciliation, chart reviews, and researching drug information questions from providers, staff, and patients, further expanding the impact of the pharmacist within the practice. In 2019, the embedded pharmacists, working two days a week on site, completed 771 in-person and phone visits, notable interventions included but were not limited to removal or addition of medication therapy (n = 85), adjustment of medication dose (n = 235), changing ineffective therapy (n = 24), adherence identification and intervention (n = 58), and patient education (n = 75).

In 2016, an embedded pharmacist position was created at the private medical group senior care clinic (SCC), enabling it to achieve a Patient-Centered Medical Home (PCMH) status. The clinic provider group, comprised of mostly seasoned practitioners, had never worked with an embedded clinical pharmacist and did not know what services could be provided outside of medication reconciliation. Through shadowing, engagement with providers, and collaboration with other PCMH-certified clinics within the SCC providers learned how other facilities across the country were utilizing embedded pharmacists to improve patient care beyond medication reconciliation. Collaborative practice agreements were developed, and the pharmacist scope was expanded to include the referral-based chronic disease state management, with a focus on reduction in documented ADRs and improved medication therapy outcomes.

Despite these advances, sustainability and expansion of the SCC embedded-pharmacy practice was limited by the ability of the pharmacist to bill for the health services provided. The ability of the pharmacist to bill for non-dispensing health services was limited by staff awareness, healthcare facility infrastructure, and supports. A portion of the pharmacist's time was subsidized by the university to support co-development and pilot testing of a billing and coding toolkit to support training and necessary coding and billing infrastructure within the EHR and facility. Over the past year, processes for submitting claims to both public and private payers have been established, over 100 claims submitted, reasons for rejected claims collected, and patient satisfaction measured.

4. Discussion

In this manuscript, we demonstrate how five practice sites approached and implemented non-dispensing pharmacy health services in the primary care setting to enhance medication adherence, improve health outcomes, and reduce the number of adverse events [29,30]. We utilized the CFIR implementation framework to identify, understand, and highlight complex multicomponent healthcare factors that influenced the implementation of embedded pharmacists within the primary care practice.

CFIR allowed researchers across sites to establish a common vernacular to facilitate systematic interventions. We identified two overarching modifiable factors that influence current and future practice delivery and highlight the role of academia as an incubator for practice change and implementation: Data collection and information sharing.

Improved Data Collection: Making a convincing argument that a pharmacist should be added to a care team may first require an objective proof that a pharmacist will add value and help meet the needs of that team. This was the case for each of our sites and became evidence as each site shared their anecdotal and/or limited data during the semi-structured interviews. Data collection grew slowly with the addition of clinical tasks and responsibilities. Initially, pharmacists consulted with providers, reviewing charts, and identifying issues, with little to no documentation of their efforts in the medical record. As the interactions between providers, pharmacists, and patients increased, documentation and collection of data increased. However, current methods of data collection at the embedded sites are onerous (with the exception of the grant funded specialty position), systems are not in place to support collection of pharmacist interventions, and make it difficult to recognize and reimburse individual providers for their contribution. Without a streamlined method to collect and differentiate contributions, it remains difficult for pharmacists to justify the need to expand the clinical services offered.

Pharmacists in many different care settings are tracking their interventions to establish the value they provide and help justify their current roles (as well as new roles). Once established, pharmacists may use intervention tracking to identify opportunities for billing. Though in some settings, these data are preliminary or significantly lacking, leaving a desire for more evidence-based practice data [31–33].

Practice-based evidence requires the collection, utilization, and sharing of available data. In order to be sustainable, data processes also need to be efficient. In our case series, we found that data collection strategies varied among practice sites and healthcare systems. To track data, some pharmacists used features of their EHR (e.g., intervention tracking in Epic), self-developed mechanisms (e.g., spreadsheet of interventions), or a mixture of both approaches. Such individual-level approaches make data aggregation, utilization, and sharing difficult. While a universally utilized, nationwide data system for pharmacists (and all healthcare practitioners) is ideal, it is unlikely to occur in the immediate future. However, it is feasible for pharmacists working in the described university system partnership to ensure consistency in data collection, which would allow for greater ease in data aggregation and cross-site comparisons.

With the difficulties in collecting data and the potentially significant time requirements, it is very important to consider what types of data should be collected and shared. Pharmacists should consider what type of activities should be recorded, what level of detail would be required, and what data would best demonstrate the value of the pharmacist/pharmacy team. Organizing interventions into categories can help narrow the focus. Some categories may include clinical care, consultations, cost savings, and patient education. The particular setting, role, and responsibilities of the pharmacist will help determine what data are collected.

To make the goal of tracking pharmacist interventions attainable, the process of recording data needs to be practical [34]. Pharmacists should ask, is there a workflow-based, efficient recording strategy I can utilize? To ensure data is efficiently recorded and adequately captured, an interface with the current software (e.g., current electronic health record) will be important. Furthermore, most pharmacists are not data experts and may require assistance from information technology personnel or those with informatics backgrounds. In future academic/clinical contracts, it may be helpful to ensure that efficient data collection is included. Standardizing data collection methods would also allow pharmacists to collaborate on research more effectively [35].

Improved Data/Information Sharing: Once substantial data are collected, the dissemination of those data to key stakeholders (health system administrators, legislators, other healthcare providers, etc.) both internally and externally is essential for continued advancement of pharmacy integration and practice transformation [1,36,37]. Currently, at all but one of our sites, work-arounds have been created to collect and share information across providers. At the one site grant funds supported data template development, form creation, and data collection. EHR templates that have been adapted from other health professional EHR templates are not linked to other patient information, efforts to collect and share information unnecessarily repeated, and note fields often used inefficiently and ineffectively communicate vital patient health information among team members. In our experience, when data are shared judiciously among team members and across interprofessional teams, it can affect and spur practice change. However, diffusion, dissemination, and implementation of published clinical research results into the practice needs to be more strategic to reach the proposed change.

Internal dissemination of pharmacy interventions and data is varied among practice sites. Stakeholders may value different information depending on the practice site and their role in the organization. Internal data are generally routed to health system administrators such as chief medical officer (CMO), chief operations officer (COO), chief executive officer (CEO), chief financial officer (CFO), quality managers, and other healthcare providers. For example, at our newest practice site, data from pharmacist interventions are routed to the director of pharmacy, who then shares this valuable information with the executive suite which includes the CMO, CFO, and COO. The CMO and COO then communicate relevant findings directly to the medical providers at a monthly staff meeting. The pharmacist attends these monthly staff meetings along with behavioral health, population health, diabetes task force, and the clinical leadership team, which has assisted in integrating the new pharmacist clinical services into the practice site. Similarly, another clinic has quarterly quality meetings in which health metrics such as the percentage of patients with controlled diabetes, hypertension, and hyperlipidemia are reported to the staff. These meetings can be an opportune time to highlight pharmacist interventions and impact on the quality of care.

Despite the significant number of health advances, a substantial gap remains between sharing of this information and resultant incorporation into the clinical practice. Strategic and proactive efforts to improve data sharing are required to facilitate adoption, scale practice change, and optimize patient care delivery. To accomplish this the right information needs to be shared with the right individuals. This can be one of the greatest challenges in external data dissemination. Careful thought must be placed on whether to pursue publication in pharmacy, medicine, or public health journals. Although the amount of pharmacist publications in major medical journals has increased over the past two decades, the amount of published systematic reviews remains lacking. This may be due to the previously mentioned challenge in standardizing data collection methods.

Data from our clinics have primarily been shared in pharmacy journals. Prior to establishing any clinical service, a pharmacist needs to be able to obtain clinical privileges or a scope of practice. Sharing how other pharmacists have done this in the past and possible examples of the scopes included can guide pharmacists attempting to implement new services. However, other key stakeholders such as physicians and health system administrators may not have exposure to these publications and thus may not as widely recognize the impact pharmacists can have on clinical outcomes and quality metrics. In the future, continued expansion of pharmacist publications to major medical journals may assist in the circulation of key findings.

5. Conclusions

Academic pharmacists can be used to support program development, expand pharmacist non-dispensing services in primary care, and ultimately serve as incubators for practice change. However, data collection and information sharing are two modifiable factors that need to be addressed to better influence current and future pharmacist practice delivery.

Author Contributions: Conceptualization, R.R., E.N., J.H., and M.B.; methodology, R.R.; validation, R.R. and C.O.; formal analysis, R.R., E.N., and A.P.; data curation, C.L., A.B., T.P., A.P., and A.J.; writing—original draft preparation, R.R., A.B., M.P., N.S., J.B., and B.P.; writing—review and editing, C.L., T.P., A.P., E.N., J.H., A.J., M.B., B.B., K.C., and C.O.; supervision, R.R.; project administration, R.R. All authors have read and agreed to the published version of the manuscript.

Funding: This research received no external funding.

Conflicts of Interest: The authors declare no conflict of interest.

References

1. Dalton, K.; Byrne, S. Role of the pharmacist in reducing healthcare costs: Current insights. *Int. Pharm. Regul. Programme* **2017**, *6*, 37–46. [CrossRef] [PubMed]
2. Duedahl, T.H.; Hansen, W.B.; Kjeldsen, L.J.; Graabæk, T. Pharmacist-led interventions improve quality of medicine-related healthcare service at hospital discharge. *Eur. J. Hosp. Pharm.* **2018**, *25*, e40–e45. [CrossRef] [PubMed]
3. Livet, M.; Haines, S.T.; Curran, G.M.; Seaton, T.L.; Ward, C.S.; Sorensen, T.D.; Roth McClurg, M. Implementation Science to Advance Care Delivery: A Primer for Pharmacists and Other Health Professionals. *Pharmacotherapy* **2018**, *38*, 490–502. [CrossRef] [PubMed]
4. Seaton, T.L. Dissemination and implementation sciences in pharmacy: A call to action for professional organizations. *Res. Soc. Adm. Pharm.* **2017**, *13*, 902–904. [CrossRef] [PubMed]
5. Draugalis, J.R.; Plaza, C.M. Preparing graduate students for teaching and service roles in pharmacy education. *Am. J. Pharm. Educ.* **2007**, *71*, 105. [CrossRef]
6. Embedding Pharmacists with Physicians | AACP. Available online: https://www.aacp.org/article/embedding-pharmacists-physicians (accessed on 25 May 2020).
7. Bansal, N.; Tai, W.-T.; Chen, L.-C. Implementation of an innovative surgical pharmacy service to improve patient outcomes-Twelve-month outcomes of the Enhanced Surgical Medicines Optimization Service. *J. Clin. Pharm. Ther.* **2019**, *44*, 904–911. [CrossRef]
8. Weir, N.M.; Newham, R.; Dunlop, E.; Bennie, M. Factors influencing national implementation of innovations within community pharmacy: A systematic review applying the Consolidated Framework for Implementation Research. *Implement. Sci.* **2019**, *14*, 21. [CrossRef]
9. Meisenberg, B.; Ness, J.; Rao, S.; Rhule, J.; Ley, C. Implementation of solutions to reduce opioid-induced oversedation and respiratory depression. *Am. J. Health Syst. Pharm.* **2017**, *74*, 162–169. [CrossRef]
10. Dissemination & Implementation Models. Available online: https://dissemination-implementation.org/ (accessed on 10 May 2020).
11. Damschroder, L.J.; Aron, D.C.; Keith, R.E.; Kirsh, S.R.; Alexander, J.A.; Lowery, J.C. Fostering implementation of health services research findings into practice: A consolidated framework for advancing implementation science. *Implement. Sci.* **2009**, *4*, 50. [CrossRef]
12. McNabb, J.; Ross, J.W.; Abriola, K.; Turley, C.; Nightingale, C.H.; Nicolau, D.P. Adherence to highly active antiretroviral therapy predicts virologic outcome at an inner-city human immunodeficiency virus clinic. *Clin. Infect. Dis.* **2001**, *33*, 700–705. [CrossRef]
13. Wagner, G.J.; Kanouse, D.E.; Koegel, P.; Sullivan, G. Adherence to HIV Antiretrovirals among Persons with Serious Mental Illness. *AIDS Patient Care STDs* **2003**, *17*, 179–186. [CrossRef] [PubMed]
14. Bangsberg, D.R.; Hecht, F.M.; Charlebois, E.D.; Zolopa, A.R.; Holodniy, M.; Sheiner, L.; Bamberger, J.D.; Chesney, M.A.; Moss, A. Adherence to protease inhibitors, HIV-1 viral load, and development of drug resistance in an indigent population. *Acquir. Immune Defic. Syndr.* **2000**, *14*, 357–366. [CrossRef] [PubMed]
15. DiMatteo, M.R.; Giordani, P.J.; Lepper, H.S.; Croghan, T.W. Patient adherence and medical treatment outcomes: A meta-analysis. *Med. Care* **2002**, *40*, 794–811. [CrossRef] [PubMed]

16. Mannheimer, S.; Friedland, G.; Matts, J.; Child, C.; Chesney, M.; Terry Beirn Community Programs for Clinical Research on AIDS. The Consistency of Adherence to Antiretroviral Therapy Predicts Biologic Outcomes for Human Immunodeficiency Virus–Infected Persons in Clinical Trials. *Clin. Infect. Dis.* **2002**, *34*, 1115–1121. [CrossRef] [PubMed]
17. Hadi, M.A.; Neoh, C.F.; Zin, R.M.; Elrggal, M.; Cheema, E. Pharmacovigilance: Pharmacists & rsquo; perspective on spontaneous adverse drug reaction reporting. *Int. Pharm. Regul. Programme* **2017**, *6*, 91–98. [CrossRef]
18. Nivya, K.; Sri Sai Kiran, V.; Ragoo, N.; Jayaprakash, B.; Sonal Sekhar, M. Systemic review on drug related hospital admissions—A pubmed based search. *Saudi Pharm. J.* **2015**, *23*, 1–8. [CrossRef]
19. Jokanovic, N.; Wang, K.N.; Dooley, M.J.; Lalic, S.; Tan, E.CK.; Kirkpatrick, C.M.; Bell, J.S. Prioritizing interventions to manage polypharmacy in Australian aged care facilities. *Res. Soc. Adm. Pharm.* **2017**, *13*, 564–574. [CrossRef] [PubMed]
20. Aagaard, L.; Strandell, J.; Melskens, L.; Petersen, P.S.G.; Hansen, E.H. Global Patterns of Adverse Drug Reactions Over a Decade: Analyses of Spontaneous Reports to VigiBase^{TM}. *Drug Saf.* **2012**, *35*, 1171–1182. [CrossRef]
21. Stausberg, J. International prevalence of adverse drug events in hospitals: An analysis of routine data from England, Germany, and the USA. *BMC Health Serv. Res.* **2014**, *14*, 125. [CrossRef]
22. Marcum, Z.A.; Handler, S.M.; Boyce, R.; Gellad, W.; Hanlon, J.T. Medication misadventures in the elderly: A year in review. *Am. J. Geriatr. Pharmacother.* **2010**, *8*, 77–83. [CrossRef]
23. Dugdale, D.C.; Epstein, R.; Pantilat, S.Z. Time and the patient-physician relationship. *J. Gen. Intern. Med.* **1999**, *14*, S34–S40. [CrossRef] [PubMed]
24. Mechanic, D.; McAlpine, D.D.; Rosenthal, M. Are Patients' Office Visits with Physicians Getting Shorter? *N. Engl. J. Med.* **2001**, *344*, 198–204. [CrossRef] [PubMed]
25. Yarnall, K.S.H.; Pollak, K.I.; Østbye, T.; Krause, K.M.; Michener, J.L. Primary Care: Is There Enough Time for Prevention? *Am. J. Public Health* **2003**, *93*, 635–641. [CrossRef] [PubMed]
26. Geraghty, E.M.; Franks, P.; Kravitz, R.L. Primary Care Visit Length, Quality, and Satisfaction for Standardized Patients with Depression. *J. Gen. Intern. Med.* **2007**, *22*, 1641–1647. [CrossRef]
27. Bressler, R.; Bahl, J.J. Principles of Drug Therapy for the Elderly Patient. *Mayo Clin. Proc.* **2003**, *78*, 1564–1577. [CrossRef]
28. Davies, E.C.; Green, C.F.; Taylor, S.; Williamson, P.R.; Mottram, D.R.; Pirmohamed, M. Adverse Drug Reactions in Hospital In-Patients: A Prospective Analysis of 3695 Patient-Episodes. *PLoS ONE* **2009**, *4*, e4439. [CrossRef]
29. Robins, L.S.; Jackson, J.E.; Green, B.B.; Korngiebel, D.; Force, R.W.; Baldwin, L.-M. Barriers and Facilitators to Evidence-based Blood Pressure Control in Community Practice. *J. Am. Board Fam. Med.* **2013**, *26*, 539–557. [CrossRef]
30. Shoemaker, S.J.; Curran, G.M.; Swan, H.; Teeter, B.S.; Thomas, J. Application of the Consolidated Framework for Implementation Research to community pharmacy: A framework for implementation research on pharmacy services. *Res. Soc. Adm. Pharm.* **2017**, *13*, 905–913. [CrossRef]
31. Segal, E.M.; Bates, J.; Fleszar, S.L.; Holle, L.M.; Kennerly-Shah, J.; Rockey, M.; Jeffers, K.D. Demonstrating the value of the oncology pharmacist within the healthcare team. *J. Oncol. Pharm. Pract.* **2019**, *25*, 1945–1967. [CrossRef]
32. Roman, C.; Edwards, G.; Dooley, M.; Mitra, B. Roles of the emergency medicine pharmacist: A systematic review. *Am. J. Health-Syst. Pharm.* **2018**, *75*, 796–806. [CrossRef]
33. Milosavljevic, A.; Aspden, T.; Harrison, J. Community pharmacist-led interventions and their impact on patients' medication adherence and other health outcomes: A systematic review. *Int. J. Pharm. Pract.* **2018**, *26*, 387–397. [CrossRef] [PubMed]
34. Karampatakis, G.D.; Ryan, K.; Patel, N.; Stretch, G. Capturing pharmacists' impact in general practice: An e-Delphi study to attempt to reach consensus amongst experts about what activities to record. *BMC Fam. Pract.* **2019**, *20*, 126. [CrossRef] [PubMed]
35. McNicol, M.; Kuhn, C.; Sebastian, S. Standardized documentation workflow within an electronic health record to track pharmacists' interventions in pediatric ambulatory care clinics. *J. Am. Pharm. Assoc.* **2019**, *59*, 410–415. [CrossRef] [PubMed]

36. Manzoor, B.S.; Cheng, W.-H.; Lee, J.C.; Uppuluri, E.M.; Nutescu, E.A. Quality of Pharmacist-Managed Anticoagulation Therapy in Long-Term Ambulatory Settings: A Systematic Review. *Ann. Pharmacother.* **2017**, *51*, 1122–1137. [CrossRef] [PubMed]
37. Benedict, A.W.; Spence, M.M.; Sie, J.L.; Chin, H.A.; Ngo, C.D.; Salmingo, J.F.; Vidaurreta, A.T.; Rashid, N. Evaluation of a Pharmacist-Managed Diabetes Program in a Primary Care Setting Within an Integrated Health Care System. *J. Manag. Care Spec. Pharm.* **2018**, *24*, 114–122. [CrossRef]

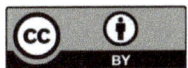

© 2020 by the authors. Licensee MDPI, Basel, Switzerland. This article is an open access article distributed under the terms and conditions of the Creative Commons Attribution (CC BY) license (http://creativecommons.org/licenses/by/4.0/).

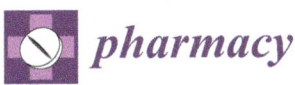

Case Report

Pilot Study: Evaluating the Impact of Pharmacist Patient-Specific Medication Recommendations for Diabetes Mellitus Therapy to Family Medicine Residents

Camlyn Masuda *, Rachel Randall and Marina Ortiz

Daniel K Inouye College of Pharmacy, University of Hawaii at Hilo, Hilo, HI 96720, USA; randall8@hawaii.edu (R.R.); ortiz33@hawaii.edu (M.O.)
* Correspondence: camlynm@hawaii.edu

Received: 4 July 2020; Accepted: 28 August 2020; Published: 31 August 2020

Abstract: Pharmacists have demonstrated effectiveness in managing diabetes mellitus (DM) and lowering hemoglobin A1C (A1C) through direct patient management. Often patients with diabetes and elevated A1C may not be able to come into the clinic for separate appointments with a pharmacist or for diabetes education classes. A novel way that pharmacists can assist in improving the control of patients' diabetes and improve prescriber understanding and the use of medications for diabetes is by providing medication recommendations to medical residents prior to the patient's appointment with the medical resident. The results of this pilot study indicate that the recommendations provided to family medicine residents and implemented at the patient's office visit helped to lower A1C levels, although the population size was too small to show statistical significance. This pilot study's results support performing a larger study to determine if the pharmacist's recommendation not only improves patient care by lowering A1C levels but if it also helps improve medical resident's understanding and use of medications for diabetes.

Keywords: chronic care management; team-based primary care; pharmacist in primary care

1. Introduction

Pharmacists in ambulatory care clinics have demonstrated effectiveness in improving the health of patients with diabetes mellitus (DM) by lowering hemoglobin A1C (A1C) [1]. A common measure of diabetes control is A1C and the American Diabetes Association (ADA) recommends lowering A1C to help prevent complications [2]. Improving management and the control of a patient's DM by lowering A1C prevents microvascular and macrovascular complications [3,4]. Sinclair et al. has shown that, in addition to improving patient care, pharmacists also help increase clinic reimbursement from value-based payments for decreasing the number of patients that have uncontrolled DM [5]. Unfortunately, pharmacists are not available in every primary care clinic and are not able to see every patient with uncontrolled DM. In addition, patients may not show up to these appointments because they have challenges getting to the clinic or are fearful to discuss their condition [6,7].

In about one-third of Family Medicine residency programs, pharmacists have been a vital member of the healthcare team and a majority of their time is spent providing pharmacotherapy recommendations [8]. To help improve the management of patients with DM and encourage the appropriate use of newer therapies (e.g., glucagon-like peptide-1 agonists) or complicated medication regimens, such as basal and bolus insulin, providing recommendations to medical residents is another way pharmacists can help improve patient care with long-term benefits. By providing these recommendations prior to a patient's appointment, the visit is enhanced by decreasing the wait time that is spent while the medical resident consults with the pharmacist and physician preceptor. The medical resident may also benefit from gaining more confidence in the appropriate use of drug therapies for DM. Medical residents come from different medical schools, which do not have consistent training in DM management and when they first start the residency program they have not had the opportunity to chronically manage severely uncontrolled patients with DM in clinic settings [9]. This pilot study was conducted to determine if pharmacist's recommendations for DM therapy in patients with A1C ≥ 8% given to family medicine residents prior to an upcoming office visit would help improve that patient's A1C levels and if these recommendations were helpful to the medical resident.

2. Materials and Methods

This was a prospective pilot, Investigational Review Board waived and privacy board approved quality improvement project conducted at the University of Hawaii at Manoa John A. Burns School of Medicine, Department of Family Medicine and Community Health clinic, located in a rural area in the state of Hawaii. The pharmacist in the clinic was employed by the University of Hawaii at Hilo Daniel K. Inouye College of Pharmacy and had a collaborative agreement and memorandum of understanding to work in the clinic. A postgraduate year one pharmacy resident also assisted with the project.

A list of patients, 18 years and older, with DM was obtained from the electronic medical record (EPIC) and stored on a secure remote desktop. The electronic medical record automatically generated this report based on diabetes mellitus diagnosis code within the office visit notes, problem list or medical history. The report calculated the percentage of patients with an A1C > 9% because this is a quality metric that is a measure of DM control and the data are reported to organizations, such as the National Committee for Quality Assurance (NCQA) and Medicare as part of the Comprehensive Primary Care Plus Program [10,11]. Although the quality metric included A1C > 9%, this study included established patients with an A1C ≥ 8% to increase the number of patients in the study and include those that had uncontrolled DM. Patients with an A1C < 8% were not selected because certain patients may have a higher target A1C goal of < 8%. ADA guidelines recommend an A1C goal of < 8% in some patients, such as those with advanced complications from diabetes (e.g., albuminuria), chronic conditions or a history of severe hypoglycemia [2].

Patients included in the pilot study were established patients, 18 years and older, with Type 2 DM, A1C ≥ 8% and had an upcoming appointment with one of the family medicine residents in the upcoming 6-8 weeks. There were no other additional exclusion criteria. Chart reviews performed on appropriate patients included researching prior DM therapies and patient-specific concerns, such as contraindications, cost, administration concerns, allergies and intolerances. Recommendations for diabetes management were patient-specific, evidence based (ADA or American Association of Clinical Endocrinologist (AACE) diabetes guidelines) [12,13] and cost effective based on patients' drug coverage. Diabetes management may be multifaceted; therefore, multiple recommendations were given per patient to encompass many possible caveats. If information in the chart did not include medical conditions that may be contraindications for use for medications, the recommendation to the medical resident included verifying with the patient if they had a history of these medical conditions. All recommendations also included medication-specific side effects to monitor. To determine the most cost-effective medications, the pharmacist reviewed the patient's drug formulary coverage on the internet whenever it was available. In addition to medication recommendations, the pharmacist also included recommendations on ordering pertinent labs (A1C, urine albumin to creatinine ratio, lipid panel, serum creatinine, etc.). The family medicine residents, who were in postgraduate training years 1-3, made the final decision to implement the recommendation based on the information obtained during the visit, which incorporated any contraindications or concerns (e.g., hypoglycemia) presented by the patient. The resident's final plan for the patient was discussed with their physician preceptor before implementation. To improve consistency of recommendations, only two pharmacists were involved in the study. A post graduate year one pharmacy resident made the initial recommendations and the supervising pharmacist, who is a certified diabetes care and education specialist, reviewed the initial recommendations and made changes to the recommendations when necessary.

The recommendations were either verbally shared with the family medicine resident, if the resident was in the clinic with the pharmacist 1–3 days before the patient's office visit, or a message was sent in the electronic medical record. Chart reviews were performed after the office visit and the following data were collected: if recommendations were accepted, if recommendations were not accepted, the reason it was not accepted and the patient's follow-up A1C drawn closest to the date of the visit. If the office visit note's assessment and plan section included the recommendation that the pharmacist provided, it was considered implemented. If the recommendation was not documented in the assessment and plan section, it was labelled as a recommendation not implemented. The rest of the office visit note was reviewed to determine reasons for lack of implementation and if no documentation of management of DM was included in the office visit note, the reason for not implementing the recommendation was labelled as not enough time to discuss DM or the patient was seen for another reason/complaint. Recommendations given to the medical residents occurred over a period of 8 weeks from June to August 2019. Changes in A1C percentage for patients that the medical resident implemented the pharmacist's recommendations (recommendation implemented) were compared to the patients that the medical resident did not implement the recommendations (recommendation not implemented) and analyzed with a paired Student's t-test. Follow-up A1C results after the office visit and the recommendation given were conducted anywhere from 2 weeks to 8 months later.

The participating family medicine residents were asked to complete a written survey. The following questions were asked: if the recommendations were helpful; if the resident wanted to continue receiving the recommendation; if they preferred receiving recommendations verbally, in writing or both.

3. Results

The original report received from the electronic medical record generated 50 unique patients. The pharmacist performed chart reviews on 27 of the 50 patients. Of the 27 patients, six patients had a baseline A1C of < 8% and were excluded from the data analysis. The pharmacist reviewed the chart and made a recommendation for DM therapy for 21 patients; 12 (57%) of the patients were male with an average age of 49 years. Only 3 patients were ≥ 65 years old. See Table 1 for additional baseline characteristics.

Table 1. Baseline Characteristics.

	All Patients Chart Reviewed ($n = 21$)	Pharmacist Recommendation Implemented ($n = 15$)	Pharmacist Recommendation Not Implemented ($n = 6$)
Age			
Between 18 and 65 years	18 (86%)	13 (87%)	5 (83%)
≥65 years	3 (14%)	2 (13%)	1 (17%)
Gender			
Female	9 (43%)	7 (47%)	2 (33%)
Male	12	8	4
Average body weight (kg)	93.4	88.6	105.3
Average baseline number of medications for diabetes	2.14	2.33	2.08
Number of patients on insulin	12	8	4

Of the 21 recommendations made, 11 (52%) were sent via electronic message in the medical record system compared to 10 (48%) conveyed to the medical resident verbally. Of those recommendations made, 15 (71%) were implemented by the medical resident. Only 6 (29%) recommendations were not implemented and the reasons for this include that patients that did not show up for their appointment ($n = 2$), patients declined recommendations ($n = 2$) and there was not enough time to discuss DM or the patient was seen for another reason/complaint ($n = 2$).

The A1C collected after the office visit was the one closest to the appointment when the pharmacist recommendation was made. In the recommendation implemented group, the follow up A1C occurred between 0.5–8 months (median 2.75 months) later, and in the recommendation not implemented group, the follow up A1C occurred between 1–3.5 months (median 1.38 months) later. There was a higher number of patients in the recommendation implemented group who had a decrease in A1C (67%) compared to the recommendation not implemented group (50%). The average difference in A1C pre and post study was decreased by 1.3% for the patients that the pharmacist's recommendation was implemented, and increased by 0.4% in the group in which the recommendation was not implemented ($p = 0.18$). Table 2 includes a comparison of the average A1C levels for all patients and the changes between groups. There were three patients in the recommendation implemented group compared to one patient in the recommendation not implemented group that did not have an A1C done after the office visit. The average A1C calculated was based on the number of patients that had an A1C available after office visit.

Table 2. Average A1C levels and change of levels.

	All Patients Chart Reviewed ($n = 21$)	Pharmacist Recommendation Implemented ($n = 15$) *	Pharmacist Recommendation Not Implemented ($n = 6$)
Effect on A1C			
A1C decreased	13 (62%)	10 (67%)	3 (50%)
A1C increased	4 (19%)	2 (13%)	2 (33%)
No A1C available	4 (19%)	3 (20%)	1 (17%)
A1C ≤ 8 post recommendation	7 (33%)	6 (40%)	1 (17%)
Average A1C prior to recommendation	10.6%	10.4%	11%
Average A1C post recommendation **	9.7%	9.1%	11.4%
Difference in A1C	−0.9%	−1.3% ($p = 0.18$)	+0.4%

* One A1C result was > 14%, which was rounded to 14% for calculating the average for the recommendation implemented group. ** Average calculated based on number of patients that had an A1C available after office visit.

Only two family medicine residents out of eleven completed the written survey (18% response rate) and all responses were that the pharmacist's recommendations were helpful, that they wanted to continue receiving the recommendations and preferred written recommendations compared to verbal.

4. Discussion

Of the patients for whom the pharmacist recommendations were implemented, a majority of patients (67%) had a decrease in their A1C, 40% of which had an A1C that was ≤ 8%, which is close to target goal of < 7% for most patients with DM [2]. The average change in A1C from pre and post recommendation decreased by 1.3% in the recommendation implemented group, whereas in the group in which recommendations were not implemented, the average A1C increased slightly (0.4%). These results indicate that pharmacist recommendations given prior to the office visit may help lower A1C levels and improve the control of DM, and are in alignment with improvements in A1C in patients being chronically managed by pharmacists compared to physician care [14]. Ambulatory care pharmacists that implement both direct patient care and provide patient-specific recommendations could help a larger number of patients with DM lower their A1C.

This study was unique in that it provided patient-specific recommendations based on clinical factors, medication history, and drug formulary coverage. A limitation of this study is that the total population was small in this pilot study, $n = 21$, and the results did not show statistical significance. One of the challenges in getting a higher number of patients in the study is the time it takes to make the patient-specific recommendations and research formulary coverage. Diabetes is a complex disease to manage and many factors, such as medication adherence and lifestyle modifications, need to be assessed before making medication changes/additions. Recommendations were made after extensive chart reviews and included caveats for use, such as assessing patient's blood glucose levels at the time of the visit, hypoglycemia and assessing if the patient had any contraindications to the medication which may not have been included in the electronic medical record. The pharmacist included many factors regarding the safety and efficacy of medications in the recommendations given and provided alternative plans if other situations occurred when the resident talked with their patient. The family medicine residents assessed the patient at the visit for any other factors that may have not been considered and made the final recommendation based on their findings from that visit. The residents also reviewed and discussed with the physician preceptor, prior to implementing the plan, which helped ensure patient safety. Thus, if there were other factors the family medicine resident obtained during the actual office visit, the recommendations were not implemented. Patients included in the study were identified by a report generated by the electronic medical record system based on the diabetes diagnosis code manually added to the record in the problem list, office visit or medical history. There were some patients with diabetes not included in the report if the physician did not enter a diabetes diagnosis code or if a patient had an incorrect primary care provider assigned to their medical record. However, this would most likely have omitted only a small number of patients.

Although the lowering of A1C is promising, there were other limitations to this study. Roughly, 19% of patients did not have an A1C drawn after their office visit or scheduled office visit, which may have influenced the average post-recommendation A1C levels. These patients did not complete lab tests or did not come in for follow up, despite recommendations and reminder calls to schedule follow up appointments. This rate is similar to average no show appointment rates of 24% reported for family practice clinics, which may indicate this is similar to real life practice [6].

ADA guidelines recommend checking an A1C every 3 months if a patient's A1C is not controlled [2]. However, in practice it is difficult to get all patients to have their A1C drawn exactly 3 months after the visit. For the purposes of this quality improvement pilot study, the A1C drawn closest to the date of the office visit where the recommendation was made ensured a consistent data point. The median of 2.75 months after the office visit for recommendations implemented is close to the recommendation to check at 3 months. However, the recommendation not implemented group's median time A1C value after the visit was 1.38 months, which may not be an appropriate comparison to the group in which the recommendation was implemented, since it was done so soon after the visit. Further analysis comparing the A1C 3 months after the recommendation versus the one done closest to the date of the office visit would be a helpful subgroup analysis to determine if the recommendations that are accepted do lower A1C, as it should be lower for both data points.

Another factor affecting post-recommendation A1C levels is adherence. Even though the family medicine resident implemented the pharmacist recommendation and prescribed new medications or altered the medication regimens, the patient may not have been compliant. Other factors, such as improper administration technique for injectable medications, although not accounted for, are worth mentioning.

This study did not create a formal protocol or treatment algorithm for the recommendations, which may cause differences in recommendations. To limit the differences, all recommendations were based on the ADA and/or AACE treatment algorithms, and a pharmacy resident provided the initial recommendation that was reviewed by one pharmacist. A protocol/treatment algorithm should be included in the larger study to ensure the consistency of recommendations as more pharmacists and pharmacy residents will be involved.

Other challenges conducting this study were duplicate pharmacist efforts made when patients rescheduled their appointment with another family medicine resident. The reasons the patient rescheduled with another resident included patient preference or that the original resident was not available (scheduled in another rotation/clinic, on vacation or sick). In these situations, the pharmacist sent the recommendation to the new family medicine resident assigned to see the patient. In some cases, the pharmacist was not aware of the change in provider until after the visit, due to last minute changes in the schedule, and the new provider did not receive the recommendation. Determining a way to link the recommendation to the patient to have it available to different family medicine residents will help to ensure the different providers have access to the recommendation.

Another objective of the study was to assess if the recommendations made by the pharmacist were helpful to the family medicine residents. Although feedback was positive and residents requested to continue receiving the recommendations, having only two surveys completed was a limitation for this part of the study. Higher survey response rates could have been achieved by distributing the survey electronically or by sending reminders the day of or the day after the visit. Supplementary studies should include survey questions that assess if the recommendations improve the residents' understanding and implementation of DM medications. Improving family medicine residents' understanding and implementation of DM medications could translate to far-reaching, long-term benefits, as this could improve therapy inertia and will further improve patient care.

Based on the promising results from this pilot, additional studies with a larger population are warranted. Additions to a future trial besides those listed above, that would improve the validity of the results, would be to add a control group, defined as those patients with DM and an A1C $\geq$ 8% that were seen by the medical residents in the same time frame but did not receive the pharmacist's recommendations.

5. Conclusions

The results of this pilot study are promising and indicate further studies are warranted to confirm that patient-specific pharmacist's recommendations for DM management given either verbally or written, to a family medicine resident prior to a patient's appointment is an effective method to reduce patient's A1C.

Author Contributions: Conceptualization, C.M.; methodology, C.M. and M.O.; validation, C.M.; formal analysis, C.M.; investigation, M.O. and C.M.; data curation, C.M.; writing—original draft preparation, C.M.; writing—review and editing, M.O. and R.R.; supervision, C.M.; project administration, C.M. and R.R. All authors have read and agreed to the published version of the manuscript.

Funding: This research received no external funding.

Acknowledgments: The research team would like to thank Jerwin Antonio, medical assistant and quality improvement specialist for assisting with obtaining reports and Desiree Navarro, clinic manager for guidance with clinic workflow. Great appreciation to Allen Chip Hixon, physician and Chair of the University of Hawaii at Manoa John A. Burns School of Medicine, Family Medicine and Community Health Department, as without his support, there would not be pharmacist presence in the Family Medicine clinic.

Conflicts of Interest: The authors declare no conflict of interest

References

1. Machado, M.; Bajcar, J.; Guzzo, G.C.; Einarson, T.R. Sensitivity of patient outcomes to pharmacist interventions. Part I: Systematic review and meta-analysis in diabetes management. *Ann. Pharmacother.* **2007**, *41*, 1569–1582. [CrossRef] [PubMed]
2. American Diabetes Association 6. Glycemic targets: Standards of medical care in diabetes—2020. *Diabetes Care* **2019**, *43*, S66–S76. [CrossRef]

3. Nathan, D.M.; A Cleary, P.; Backlund, J.-Y.C.; Genuth, S.M.; Lachin, J.M.; Orchard, T.J.; Raskin, P.; Zinman, B. Diabetes control and complications trial/epidemiology of diabetes interventions and complications (DCCT/EDIC) study research group intensive diabetes treatment and cardiovascular disease in patients with type 1 diabetes. *New Engl. J. Med.* **2005**, *353*, 2643–2653. [CrossRef] [PubMed]
4. Holman, R.R.; Paul, S.; Bethel, M.A.; Matthews, D.R.; Neil, H.A.W. 10-year follow-up of intensive glucose control in type 2 diabetes. *New Engl. J. Med.* **2008**, *359*, 1577–1589. [CrossRef]
5. Sinclair, J.; Bentley, O.S.; Abubakar, A.; Rhodes, L.A.; Marciniak, M.W. Impact of a pharmacist in improving quality measures that affect payments to physicians. *J. Am. Pharm. Assoc.* **2019**, *59*, S85–S90. [CrossRef]
6. Moore, C.G.; Wilson-Witherspoon, P.; Probst, J.C. Time and money: Effects of no-shows at a family practice residency clinic. *Fam. Med* **2001**, *33*, 6.
7. Lacy, N.L.; Paulman, A.; Reuter, M.D.; Lovejoy, B. Why We Don't Come: Patient Perceptions on No-Shows. *Ann. Fam. Med.* **2004**, *2*, 541–545. [CrossRef] [PubMed]
8. Ables, A.Z.; Baughman, O.L. The clinical pharmacist as a preceptor in a family practice residency training program. *Fam. Med.* **2002**, *34*, 5.
9. Amori, R.E.; Simon, B. A primer on diabetes mellitus: Foundations for the incoming first-year resident. *MedEdPORTAL* **2016**, *12*, 10469. [CrossRef] [PubMed]
10. "Comprehensive Diabetes Care," NCQA. Available online: https://www.ncqa.org/hedis/measures/comprehensive-diabetes-care/ (accessed on 28 April 2020).
11. Medicare CPCP Plus Quality Report 2019. Available online: https://innovation.cms.gov/files/x/cpcplus-qualrptpy2019.pdf (accessed on 28 April 2020).
12. American Diabetes Association 9. Pharmacologic approaches to glycemic treatment: Standards of medical care in diabetes—2019. *Diabetes Care* **2018**, *42*, S90–S102. [CrossRef]
13. Garber, A.J.; Abrahamson, M.J.; Barzilay, J.I.; Blonde, L.; Bloomgarden, Z.T.; Bush, M.A.; Dagogo-Jack, S.; DeFronzo, R.A.; Einhorn, D.; Fonseca, V.A.; et al. Consensus statement by the American Association of Clinical Endocrinologists and American College of Endocrinology on the comprehensive type 2 diabetes management algorithm—2019 executive summary. *Endocr. Pr.* **2019**, *25*, 69–100. [CrossRef] [PubMed]
14. Schultz, J.L.; Horner, K.E.; McDanel, D.L.; Miller, M.L.; Beranek, R.L.; Jacobsen, R.B.; Sly, N.J.; Miller, A.C.; A Mascardo, L. Comparing clinical outcomes of a pharmacist-managed diabetes clinic to usual physician-based care. *J. Pharm. Pr.* **2017**, *31*, 268–271. [CrossRef] [PubMed]

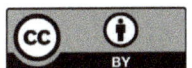

© 2020 by the authors. Licensee MDPI, Basel, Switzerland. This article is an open access article distributed under the terms and conditions of the Creative Commons Attribution (CC BY) license (http://creativecommons.org/licenses/by/4.0/).

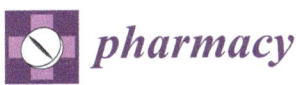

Case Report

From Pilot to Scale, the 5 Year Growth of a Primary Care Pharmacist Model

Jordan Spillane * and Erika Smith

Froedtert & The Medical College of Wisconsin, Wauwatosa, WI 53226, USA; erika.smith@froedtert.com
* Correspondence: jordan.spillane@froedtert.com; Tel.: +26-253-251-67

Received: 23 June 2020; Accepted: 25 July 2020; Published: 30 July 2020

Abstract: This case report details the five year journey of implementing, growing and optimizing a primary care pharmacist model in the ambulatory clinic setting within a health system. There is published evidence supporting the numerous benefits of including pharmacists in the primary care medical team model. This case report provides information regarding evolution of practice, the pharmacists' roles, justification and financial models for the pharmacist services, as well as lessons learned and determined conclusions.

Keywords: ambulatory pharmacy; practice growth; academic medical center; innovative practice

1. Introduction

Over the past decade, health systems have undergone dramatic changes to meet the need for improved quality of care and outcomes. Health systems are now focused on the quadruple aim: enhancing patient experience, improving population health, reducing costs, and improving the work–life balance of health care providers [1]. In the ambulatory clinic setting, new strategies have stressed the importance of team-based, patient centered care that focuses not only on clinical outcomes but also on patient experience and financial implications [2]. Clinical pharmacists are in a unique position to be an essential member of this changing landscape and can provide effective collaboration to target the quadruple aim [3].

Multiple studies have shown the significant impact pharmacists can make to improve the quality of care and outcomes. In one large integrated health care system, pharmacists providing medication therapy management (MTM) services had an estimated return on investment (ROI) of $1.29 per $1 spent, while 95.3% of patients agreed or strongly agreed that their overall health had improved because of MTM [4]. Pharmacists have also shown benefit in several chronic disease states. For patients with atrial fibrillation, MTM services decreased emergency department visits, hospitalizations, and annual total care costs [5]. For patients with end stage renal disease, pharmacist interventions are estimated to save $3.98 for every $1 spent on pharmaceutical care [6]. For patients with uncomplicated mental health conditions, ambulatory care pharmacists supported an average decrease in PHQ-9 scores from 14.5 to 8.5 [7].

The American Society of Health System Pharmacists (ASHP) has the firm belief that pharmacists are vital in providing primary care [8]. With a 22% decline in primary care physicians, ASHP believes pharmacists can be utilized to improve access and continuity in care while contributing to chronic disease state management [8,9]. In addition, studies have shown that other medical professions are supportive of pharmacists in primary care settings. In a Likert survey (scale of 1–5) given to physicians and nurses who work with clinical pharmacists at an ambulatory cancer center, the response was overwhelmingly positive with median scores of 5 on questions such as the pharmacist had a positive impact and improved outcomes, the pharmacist allowed the clinic to run more efficiently, and a full time pharmacist in clinic would be valuable [10]. Throughout the country, health systems have implemented models that allow pharmacists to order laboratory tests, initiate or modify medications and educate patients with the goal of improving the quality of care that patients receive [8].

This case report describes one health system's experience with the evolution of primary care pharmacist's service scope, utilization, and outcomes from part-time pilot to scale. It is important to note the other contributing factors to the success of this journey including the health system growth, specifically a group practice physician strategy, evolving payer mix, and competitive landscape.

Froedtert Health comprises eastern Wisconsin's only academic medical center, five hospitals, nearly 2000 physicians and more than 40 health centers and clinics. The health system represents the collaboration between Wisconsin's largest multispecialty physician practice with two community-based physician groups. In the most recent fiscal year, outpatient visits exceeded 1.3 million, inpatient admissions were 52,855 and visits to the network physicians totaled 1,059,268.

2. Evolution of Primary Care Pharmacy

As the health system's group practice strategy evolved so did the concept of leveraging the pharmacist. The ambulatory pharmacy department started at Froedtert Hospital, the academic medical center, in 1996 with a part time Anticoagulation Clinic created to address patient safety in relation to high risk medication management, as well as improve provider satisfaction. The model of the ambulatory pharmacy department has subsequently grown to support both specialty focused clinics and primary care. In this model, ambulatory clinic pharmacists develop collaborative practice agreements (CPA's) that describe the disease states, medication classes, and labs that can be reviewed and ordered by the pharmacist. In Wisconsin, the law regarding the pharmacist's scope of practice is broad and allows for physician delegation. In 2007, the organization identified a strategy to improve clinical education provided to its primary care affiliated clinics, while at the same time reducing the presence of pharmaceutical representatives in the clinic. The pharmacy department was asked to develop and support an unbiased provider education model around medications. This initiative started as twice-monthly educational sessions provided in person by pharmacists at four clinics. As the primary care site footprint grew from four to nine over a one-year period, this strategy evolved into virtual learning sessions (via teleconference) and the contracted FTE between primary care and pharmacy was re-evaluated. A pilot model of leveraging two part time pharmacists sharing time at four clinic sites was developed. This model included embedding the pharmacist physically at their clinic sites for $\frac{1}{2}$ to 1 full day per week. The four largest sites were chosen to receive this support. Key outcome measures included drug therapy consults, cost savings, and therapeutic interchange initiatives. Over time, it also evolved to focusing on patients transitioning from the inpatient environment back to their primary care physician (PCP).

The model of part-time pharmacist support struggled in terms of proving concrete outcomes, as there was no specific disease state area of focus. It also proved to be challenging for the pharmacists to become a reliable member of the care team with such limited hours of support. Thus, the model evolved to a one-year pilot using one full time pharmacist splitting time 50/50 with two of the largest primary care clinics. A key component to the success of this second model was the pharmacist that was hired for this role had experience in establishing new services and working in a fully capitated health system supporting primary care clinical outcomes. The primary care pharmacist model quickly began to focus on outcome and cost based metrics with an emphasis on diabetes and inpatient transitions of care. Because of this focus, during a time when the health system was also starting its journey towards taking on financial risk with payer partners, the model was able to show demonstrable results for an outcome where there was already financial incentives. After a year, this pharmacist model was brought forward for executive leadership discussion and a second pharmacist FTE was approved. This pharmacist was positioned to focus on and support the newly formed Care Coordination department and shared risk goals. The concept of embedding a pharmacist within Care Coordination was felt to be a reasonable next iterative step towards scaling pharmacist support across the growing group practice locations.

In 2015, the health system formed a unified group practice of three legacy physician practices. This increased the number of disparate primary care sites from approximately 10 to 25. Senior leadership that led this new group practice identified the need for a pharmacy leader on their executive team and the pharmacy leader with the most ambulatory experience was chosen. This allowed for a deep shared understanding of the goals and strategies for both group practice success and ambulatory pharmacy expansion. The Chief Medical Officer (CMO) of the group practice also had a role in leading the population health strategies of the organization. By having a strong relationship with the CMO, the pharmacy leader was able to be at the forefront of developing population health strategies.

One area of focus was concerning patients with uncontrolled diabetes. Pharmacists providing diabetes care in ambulatory settings has been shown to decrease hemoglobin A1c, systolic blood pressure, and low-density lipoprotein cholesterol [11]. As a result, in 2016, a population health approach to managing uncontrolled type 2 diabetics (A1c > 9%) was formed and called the Ambulatory Diabetes Outreach Program (ADOP). This program included leveraging the two existing pharmacist FTE, as well as adding 1 FTE pharmacist and 1 FTE Certified Diabetes Educator (CDE) RN. This was the health system's first step to proactive population based outreach and enrollment in a care team providing virtual support and disease state management to patients via telephone. The first patient population enrolled was the covered lives for which the health system had taken on some financial risk. The population health approach also included a strategy to integrate digital technologies to augment care by improving patient engagement in their healthcare. This strategy aligned with the health system's investment in the formation of a new digital health accelerator company, and positioned ambulatory pharmacy as a key collaborator willing to work towards shared goals.

The primary care pharmacists were embedded in assigned clinics as much as possible with time present matching to clinic size, while the CDE RN focused support of the centralized care coordination department. Pharmacists also maintained provider-referred patients for other disease states including hypertension and polypharmacy. Having the specific population focus of the uncontrolled type 2 diabetic population (via the ADOP initiative) helped articulate the role and scope for the smaller sites with less historical exposure to pharmacist services.

Over the next 3 years, the demand for expansion and broadening of the primary care pharmacist model led to approval of an additional four FTE of primary care pharmacists. The program demonstrated a significant improvement in diabetes specific outcome goals, as well as broad patient and provider acceptance and demand.

3. Initial Lessons Learned

As alluded to above, having a pharmacy leader fully embedded in the group practice executive leadership team led to incredible insight and creative application of pharmacy support services beyond the typical primary care pharmacist role. This helped build trust and shared accountability in positioning the goal of a successful embedded primary care pharmacist program as something that multiple stakeholders had an interest in, such as group practice operations, population health/clinically integrated network, innovation and digital therapeutics. When opportunities arose, such as changes leading to access constraints in one market, the primary care pharmacist was thought of as a potential solution alongside advanced practice providers by the Chief Operating Officer (COO) of the group practice.

Consistency in the model of primary care pharmacist deployment is ultimately necessary. There are several options to consider for the primary care pharmacist model: centralized with no co-location at clinics, clinic attribution with minimal co-location, or site attribution with majority co-location. In each of the models, consistency must be maintained via a central pharmacy leader and intentional workload prioritization determined by pharmacy and senior clinic leadership. There are positives and negatives with each model (see Table 1). One key benefit of an embedded pharmacist model is that it allows for easier patient visit access and being potentially leveraged to avoid unnecessary physician visit utilization. The VA health system has optimized this model and subsequently changed both physician and patient expectations of whom and how their care is managed [12]. They have seen success with these changes resulting in increases in both number and scope of ambulatory pharmacists at VA systems [13]. One potential downside of embedding is that the pharmacist can be pulled into non-top of license broader care team work more easily. Within the centrally located model, the pharmacist can be successful with early adopter physicians who are open to collaboration with an extended care team member. Communication with various physicians can be more challenging in the centrally located model and can seem more onerous to the provider not having easy access face to face with the pharmacist. Lastly, splitting time amongst a high number of clinics and being primarily centrally located limits the pharmacist's ability to be easily accessible for patient visits.

Table 1. Pros/Cons with Pharmacist Models.

	Pros	Cons
Embedded Pharmacists Model	Easier patient visit access Can help avoid unnecessary physician visit utilization Proven to be effective and successful in several publications Better patient outcomes, patient satisfaction, better efficiency, etc. Streamlined face-to-face communication with providers Easier integration into care teams Improved transitions of care Can increase job satisfaction	Pharmacists must ensure their work is at the top of their education and training Logistics (i.e.,: physical space, clinic staff support) need to be determined
Centrally Located Model	Less disruptive to workflow within clinic Can streamline communication between pharmacists & leadership Improved equity amongst pharmacists	Communication with providers can be less efficient May take more time to create positive and trusting relationships with providers Workflows are necessary for appropriately scheduling pharmacist visits Model may be more reliant on the provider actively connecting the patient to the pharmacist

Conclusion: Ultimately, the embedded model was chosen due to its ability to allow for stronger relationship building with the care team, easier integration into providing care to patients, and better real time access for patient visits.

In this health system, the model that has demonstrated the most success is clinic attributed embedded pharmacists aligned with an appropriate number of clinics based on patient volume/panel size, and with a clear population focus to align their services with the organization's strategic goals. The embedded pharmacist allows for stronger relationship building with the providers and care teams, easier integration into patient care and better real time access for patient visits. Having these established relationships has also allowed for more facile development of new services, testing of new models, and quicker provider acceptance of patient care decisions made by the pharmacist.

4. Primary Care Pharmacist Roles

The pharmacist role in primary care and population health is to achieve valued outcomes for patients, as well as organizational goals. To accomplish this, the pharmacists provide care to patients that are referred by the physician or they proactively contact patients that match certain health metrics. The primary care pharmacists focus on both routine chronic disease state management services (diabetes, hypertension, polypharmacy/complex medication regimen review) and predetermined populations (i.e., diabetic patients with A1c >9, uncontrolled hypertensive patients on 2 or more blood pressure medications). This model recognizes the importance of the relationship between the patient and primary care physician, while also layering on services from the extended care team to selected uncontrolled populations without requiring the physician to determine that the patient needs additional support. The selected populations can be prioritized and evolve over time to align with patient, provider and organization need. These can include patients with select uncontrolled disease states, or there could be specific work done with a broader look at the patient's various uncontrolled healthcare gaps, or include a medication specific focus such as safety initiatives or medication de-prescribing efforts.

Primary care pharmacists are leveraged as a resource to help in the ongoing education of providers and care teams. The primary care pharmacists write and circulate an electronic monthly newsletter of primary care focused topics, including guideline updates, primary care literature evaluations, and new drug approvals. Additionally, the pharmacists provide clinical presentations every quarter at the provider meetings across all the primary care health centers. This has been greatly appreciated by the providers and has helped remind all of the important role the pharmacists play as part of the clinic team. A primary care pharmacist is a member of the Ambulatory Therapeutics Committee and co-chaired a workgroup that focused on improving the safety and accuracy with administering vaccines across all clinics. The primary care pharmacists have been educated on the retail pharmacy services that the organization provides and have created positive working relationships with the retail pharmacists. This has helped the primary care pharmacists feel confident in recommending these services to their patients, which decreases the risk of polypharmacy, improves the rate of medication adherence and provides revenue to the organization.

5. Justification of Services

In order to maintain and optimize the primary care pharmacist model, it is very important to have access to data and communicate the benefits consistently to senior clinic leadership and physicians. In regards to the data, it is essential that an efficient and standardized workflow is created for the pharmacists to follow. This allows for the electronic health record to be optimized and provide data without requiring manual manipulation. A monthly dashboard of productivity and quality metrics was created and is shared with the primary care pharmacists on a monthly basis, and shared with the physicians and senior clinic leadership on a less frequent yet consistent basis. The dashboard can be drilled down to the individual pharmacist, which is shared by the pharmacy leader 1 on 1 with each pharmacist. This data helps the pharmacists feel confident in their clinical decisions and workflows, while also helping them determine what needs to be further refined to improve their individualized metrics. Based on these metrics and reviews of other primary care pharmacist models, a patient panel size was determined for each primary care pharmacist. This expectation was shared with the pharmacists and is reviewed on a monthly basis to hold each pharmacist accountable. Because the pharmacists are co-located at the clinics a majority of time, it is essential for the pharmacy leader to create a positive, virtual working relationship with each pharmacist. This typically involves face-to-face regular meetings at the start of the working relationship and demonstrated consistency with following-up on email communications. After the trusting relationship has been formed, having effective virtual meetings has proven to be successful. It is also essential that the pharmacist create strong working relationships with their providers, clinic staff and local clinic leadership. Finally, an important factor that should not be overlooked in ensuring success with this model is encouraging the physicians to talk to their patients about the role of the pharmacist in their care. The pharmacists have found that patients are more likely to agree to work with the primary care pharmacists and ultimately achieve better care outcomes when this warm hand off occurs.

6. Financial Models

There are several considerations in relation to the financial model to support expansion of primary care pharmacist services. The lack of provider status for pharmacists and subsequent inability to bill for clinical services provided by the pharmacists requires health systems to be creative to justify primary care pharmacist services. There are several options that allow for primary care pharmacists to provide clinical services without requiring the health system to incur the full expense of the FTE.

School of Pharmacy faculty funding support is an option that can provide a portion of a primary care pharmacist FTE to provide care in the ambulatory setting without requiring a significant financial investment from the organization. With this option, it is important to ensure the partnership with the School of Pharmacy allows for alignment of the faculty pharmacists model of care with what the organization has deemed as value added. Additionally, pharmacy residency training has expanded significantly, especially PGY2 ambulatory focused residencies, which has grown by 112% over the last five years [14]. By having PGY2 ambulatory focused residents, additional primary care pharmacy services can be provided at a significantly reduced financial rate.

There are other options that increase revenue for the organization to help with off-setting the expense of the primary care pharmacist FTE. Because pharmacists do not have provider status, it is essential to have positive working relationships with Compliance, Risk, IT and Finance representatives within the organization. This allows for optimization of reimbursement through compliant channels for the primary care pharmacists. In the non-hospital clinic space, pharmacists have minimal billing opportunities and primarily bill incident-to the provider. Billing incident-to requires direct supervision of the provider (must be located in the same clinic suite) at the time that the pharmacist is providing service to the patient and also has specific documentation requirements. While reimbursement is very minimal when billing incident-to in the professional setting, it is often helpful to demonstrate any incremental revenue, along with cost savings, to the organization. Payers may be interested in piloting a program where primary care pharmacists are paid for their patient encounters while being held accountable to shared clinical expectations and total cost of care reduction. If a strategic goal is to improve patient access to providers, pharmacists can provide certain visits to allow for physicians to focus on visits requiring diagnosis or complicated disease state management. Prescription revenue associated with utilization of the organization's retail pharmacies is another way to tie actual dollars into support of pharmacy services. Other options focus on saving costs for the organization. Fully at risk organizations have a closely managed medication formulary for both in clinic administration as well as outpatient prescribing. Clinic based pharmacists have typically been very involved in the assessment and roll out of these initiatives leading to cost savings for their organizations [15,16]. And last but certainly not least, the continual growth of technology in support of efficient, evidence based care for populations will have significant impact on how the primary care practice of the future looks. Automation of appropriate patient care activities and stratification of populations that need additional management will continue to allow all care team members to operate more efficiently, including pharmacists.

Several of the above financial models have demonstrated success within the health system. The strong partnership with the Medical College of Wisconsin School of Pharmacy has allowed for additional FTE to provide pharmacy services in the primary care clinics, while also providing an excellent learning APPE experience to several learners. The health system has three PGY2 ambulatory pharmacy residents who complete a longitudinal primary care rotation, which allows for an entire additional 1.0 FTE to provide pharmacy services either through the residents' staffing or by allowing additional capacity for the preceptors throughout the second half of the residency year. The majority of the primary care clinics are located in the professional space, so incident-to billing is utilized by the pharmacists when appropriate. Although this revenue is not significant, it is direct revenue correlated to the pharmacists' services. When reviewing revenue from prescription capture, it is essential to have the data capabilities to drill down to the detailed level to determine how the primary care pharmacists are positively impacting this. The pharmacists have allowed for perceived increased access to the primary care providers by providing intensive focus on uncontrolled diabetes and optimizing hypertension medications without requiring PCP office visits.

7. Conclusions

Over the past 5 years, the primary care pharmacist team has grown from 1 FTE covering two primary care clinics to 7 FTE plus 3 PGY2 pharmacy residents covering all 25 primary care clinics. Determination for the appropriate scale for this innovative team is based on number of providers, provider panel sizes and the individual pharmacist's panel size. A lot of work has occurred on implementing, maintaining and optimizing the organization's current primary care pharmacist model. More work needs to continue in order to effectively grow this model. As previously stated, the ability to quantify how a pharmacist can improve physician access or increase their patient panel is important to the organization. An area of focus for the upcoming year is to create a definition of appropriate pharmacist utilization and calculate the associated financial outcomes related to that. It is important for pharmacy leadership to be aware of changes to the organization or payer landscape so that growth can occur in accordance with those changes. As quality metrics or shared risk models continue to grow in importance to the organization, it is essential to creatively think about how primary care pharmacists can impact those metrics effectively and efficiently.

It cannot be understated as to how important it is to share clinical data and successes of the primary care pharmacist model with the pharmacists, providers, clinic and senior leadership. The majority of the clinical data results for these primary care pharmacists is related to the uncontrolled type 2 diabetes patient population. All key stakeholders need to be consistently reminded of the positives and successes of the primary care pharmacist model. This will help with maintaining, as well as growing the model. The more people who understand what the pharmacists are capable of producing within clinic practice, the more success will be seen and pharmacists will be sought after to solve appropriate problems.

For some organizations, senior leaders and physicians, the primary care pharmacist model can be a new endeavor. The pharmacy leader will have a lot of heavy lifting to do while requesting and implementing this model. Relationships of the pharmacy team with others outside of pharmacy are key to the success of creating such a program. These relationships span all roles and disciplines across the organization. It is particularly helpful to understand what is most important to the key stakeholders so that data can center on that and be shared appropriately. It is also incredibly helpful to network with innovative ambulatory pharmacists and leaders outside of the organization to understand creative models and best practices. The pharmacy leader must demonstrate accountability by sharing both successes, as well as challenges and failures with the model. This case review documents the steps that were taken, primarily over a five year period, to request, implement, optimize, maintain and effectively plan for future growth of a primary care pharmacist model at a health system.

Author Contributions: Conceptualization, J.S. and E.S.; writing—original draft preparation, J.S. and E.S.; writing—review and editing, J.S., E.S. All authors have read and agreed to the published version of the manuscript.

Funding: This research received no external funding.

Acknowledgments: Thank you to Medical College of Wisconsin School of Pharmacy for providing support in the writing of this case report.

Conflicts of Interest: The authors declare no conflict of interest.

References

1. Bodenheimer, T.; Sinsky, C. From triple to quadruple aim: Care of the patient requires care of the provider. *Ann. Fam. Med.* **2014**, *12*, 573–576. [CrossRef] [PubMed]
2. American College of Clinical Pharmacy; McBane, S.E.; Dopp, A.L.; Abe, A.; Benavides, S.; Chester, E.A.; Dixon, D.L.; Dunn, M.; Johnson, M.; Nigro, S.J.; et al. Collaborative drug therapy management and comprehensive medication management—2015. *Pharmacother. J. Hum. Pharmacol. Drug Ther.* **2015**, *35*, e39–e50. [CrossRef]
3. Hager, K.; Murphy, C.; Uden, D.; Sick, B. Pharmacist-physician collaboration at a family medicine residency program: A focus group study. *Innov. Pharm.* **2018**, *9*, 9. [CrossRef]
4. De Oliveira, D.R.; Brummel, A.R.; Miller, D.B. Medication therapy management: 10 years of experience in a large integrated health care system. *J. Manag. Care Pharm.* **2010**, *16*, 185–195. [CrossRef]
5. Jones, L.K.; Greskovic, G.; Grassi, D.M.; Graham, J.; Sun, H.; Gionfriddo, M.R.; Murray, M.F.; Manickam, K.; Nathanson, D.C.; Wright, E.A.; et al. Medication therapy disease management: Geisinger's approach to population health management. *Am. J. Health Pharm.* **2017**, *74*, 1422–1435. [CrossRef] [PubMed]
6. Manley, H.J.; Carroll, C.A. The clinical and economic impact of pharmaceutical care in end-stage renal disease patients. *Semin. Dial.* **2002**, *15*, 45–49. [CrossRef] [PubMed]
7. Herbert, C.; Winkler, H. Impact of a clinical pharmacist–managed clinic in primary care mental health integration at a Veterans Affairs health system. *Ment. Health Clin.* **2018**, *8*, 105–109. [CrossRef] [PubMed]
8. American Society of Health System Pharmacists. ASHP statement on the pharmacist's role in primary care. *Am. J. Health Pharm.* **1999**, *56*, 1665–1667. [CrossRef] [PubMed]

9. Heilmann, R.M.F.; Campbell, S.; A Kroner, B.; Proksel, J.R.; Billups, S.J.; Witt, D.M.; Helling, D.K. Evolution, current structure, and role of a primary care clinical pharmacy service in an integrated managed care organization. *Ann. Pharmacother.* **2013**, *47*, 124–131. [CrossRef] [PubMed]
10. A Randolph, L.; Walker, C.K.; Nguyen, A.T.; Zachariah, S.R. Impact of pharmacist interventions on cost avoidance in an ambulatory cancer center. *J. Oncol. Pharm. Pract.* **2016**, *24*, 3–8. [CrossRef] [PubMed]
11. Fazel, M.T.; Bagalagel, A.; Lee, J.K.; Martin, J.; Slack, M.K. Impact of diabetes care by pharmacists as part of health care team in ambulatory settings: A systematic review and meta-analysis. *Ann. Pharmacother.* **2017**, *51*, 890–907. [CrossRef] [PubMed]
12. Galewitz, P. Clinical pharmacists employed by VA have increased nearly 50% in 5 years. *Pharm. Today* **2017**, *23*, 6–7. [CrossRef]
13. Cone, S.M.; Brown, M.C.; Stambaugh, R.L. Characteristics of ambulatory care clinics and pharmacists in Veterans Affairs medical centers: An update. *Am. J. Health Pharm.* **2008**, *65*, 631–635. [CrossRef] [PubMed]
14. ASHP 2019 Residency Match Phase I Shows Continued Increase in Positions. Available online: https://www.ashp.org (accessed on 4 June 2020). Published 15 March 2019.
15. Debenito, J.M.; Billups, S.J.; Tran, T.S.; Price, L.C. Impact of a clinical pharmacy anemia management service on adherence to monitoring guidelines, clinical outcomes, and medication utilization. *J. Manag. Care Pharm.* **2014**, *20*, 715–720. [CrossRef] [PubMed]
16. Britt, R.B.; Hashem, M.G.; Bryan, W.E.; Kothapalli, R.; Brown, J.N. Economic outcomes associated with a pharmacist-adjudicated formulary consult service in a veterans affairs medical center. *J. Manag. Care Spéc. Pharm.* **2016**, *22*, 1051–1061. [CrossRef] [PubMed]

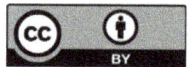

© 2020 by the authors. Licensee MDPI, Basel, Switzerland. This article is an open access article distributed under the terms and conditions of the Creative Commons Attribution (CC BY) license (http://creativecommons.org/licenses/by/4.0/).

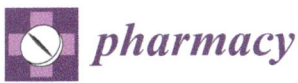

Case Report

Trends in Clinical Pharmacist Integration in Family Medicine Residency Programs in North America

Jennie B. Jarrett [1],* and Jody L. Lounsbery [2]

1 Department of Pharmacy Practice, Chicago College of Pharmacy, University of Illinois, Chicago, IL 60612, USA
2 Department of Pharmaceutical Care & Health Systems, College of Pharmacy, University of Minnesota, Minneapolis, MN 55455, USA; loun0015@umn.edu
* Correspondence: jarrett8@uic.edu

Received: 16 June 2020; Accepted: 22 July 2020; Published: 24 July 2020

Abstract: (1) **Objective**: To determine the change in prevalence of clinical pharmacists as clinician educators within family medicine residency programs (FMRPs) in North America and to describe their clinical, educational and administrative scope over time. (2) **Methods**: A systematic review of the literature was performed starting with an electronic search of PubMed and Embase for articles published between January 1980 and December 2019. Studies were included if they surveyed clinical pharmacists regarding their clinical, educational, or other roles in FMRPs in the United States or Canada. The primary outcome was the change in prevalence of clinical pharmacists in North America. Secondary outcomes included: demographic information of clinical pharmacists, change in the prevalence in Canada and United States, and descriptions of clinical services, educational roles, and other activities of clinical pharmacists within FMRPs. (3) **Results**: Of the 65 articles identified, six articles met the inclusion criteria. The prevalence of clinical pharmacists as clinician educators in FMRPs in North America has grown from 24% to 53% in the United States (U.S.) and from 14% to 47% in Canada over the study period. The clinical and educational roles are similar including: the direct patient care, clinical education, and interprofessional education and practice. (4) **Conclusion**: The prevalence of clinical pharmacists in FMRPs is growing across North America. Clinical pharmacists are highly educated and trained to support these clinician educator positions. While educational roles are consistent, clinical pharmacists' patient care roles are unique to their clinical site and growing.

Keywords: pharmacist; medical education; family medicine; graduate medical education; interprofessional

1. Introduction

The American College of Clinical Pharmacy outlined eight standards of practice for clinical pharmacists, including qualifications, process of care, documentation, collaborative team-based practice and privileging, professional development and the maintenance of competence, professionalism and ethics, research and scholarship, and other responsibilities. These other responsibilities may include the roles of educators, clinical preceptors, mentors, administrators, and policy developers. Based on these standards, clinical pharmacists are educated and trained professionals who work in direct patient care environments. Clinical pharmacists use a patient care framework, the Pharmacist Patient Care Process, to identify, assess, evaluate, and monitor patients' medication-related needs. Clinical pharmacists collaborate directly with other healthcare professionals to provide care for patients [1,2]. Within training programs like family medicine residency programs (FMRPs), clinical pharmacists have the opportunity to display their role as clinician educators. Clinical educators are practitioners who are also dedicated to teaching and developing themselves as educators [3].

Clinical pharmacists have been clinician educators in family medicine residency programs (FMRPs) for several decades, with the first account of their roles documented in 1977 [4]. Clinical pharmacists' roles within FMRPs have been further described, and family medicine physician perceptions of their integration in both the United States and Canada have been positive. Physicians reported having clinical pharmacists integrated into their practices which resulted in positive effects on patient care, meaningful contributions to knowledge, and an increased understanding of interprofessional team practices [5–9].

Pharmacy education and training in North America has evolved over the past several decades to support direct patient care, interprofessional education, and collaborative practices. The latest standards in the United States from the Accreditation Council for Pharmacy Education incorporates the Institute of Medicine recommendations for the education of all healthcare professionals [10]. Attributes these pharmacists should possess upon graduation include competencies to meet the needs of contemporary practice such as: provide patient-centered care, work in interprofessional teams, employ evidence-based practices, apply quality improvement methods, and use informatics [11]. The most recent standards from the Canadian Council's Accreditation of Pharmacy Programs also mirror these competencies [12]. Post-graduate pharmacy residency training in both the United States and Canada embrace these competencies as well to train pharmacy graduates in the additional skills necessary for these unique patient care and educational positions [13–15]. This shift in focus to address the needs of contemporary practices, including interprofessional education and collaborative practices, has likely influenced the role of the clinical pharmacist within FMRPs.

The primary objective of this review is to determine the change in prevalence of clinical pharmacists as clinician educators in FMRPs in North America over time. The secondary objective was to describe the clinical, educational, and administrative scope of these clinical pharmacists in FMRPs.

2. Materials and Methods

This systematic review was performed in accordance with the preferred reporting items for systematic reviews and meta-analyses (PRISMA) guidance [16].

A researcher (J.L.L.) conducted an electronic search of PubMed and Embase for articles published between January 1980 and December 2019. The search was completed on 8 May 2020. Searches included keywords of the following terms: *family medicine residency, family practice residency, pharmacist*, and *pharmacy*. Broad terms, such as family medicine residency, were combined in strings with specific terms, such as pharmacist, for focused results. Search results were limited to the English language. Bibliographies of the included articles were reviewed for potential additional articles for meeting the criteria for inclusion.

Studies were included in this review if they surveyed clinical pharmacists regarding their clinical, educational, or other roles in FMRPs in the United States or Canada. Studies were excluded if: (1) only abstracts could be obtained via library access at either the University of Minnesota or University of Illinois at Chicago; (2) the survey related to an intervention-based project or service; (3) the survey was not conducted nationally across either the U.S. or Canada; (4) it was not within an FMRP. Article citations and abstracts were downloaded into a text document for review. Authors (J.B.J. and J.L.L.) performed title and abstract screening independently. The title and abstract screening results were discussed between the authors (J.B.J. and J.L.L.) and inclusion/exclusion discrepancies were determined through consensus.

The primary outcome was the change in prevalence of clinical pharmacists in North America. Secondary outcomes included: the demographic information of clinical pharmacists, change in prevalence in Canada and the United States, and descriptions of clinical service, educational roles, and other activities of clinical pharmacists within FMRPs.

Descriptive statistics were used to calculate quantitative data not described explicitly by the study authors. A chi-squared statistical test was performed to determine the changes in prevalence of clinical pharmacists in FMRPs in the U.S. and Canada. A thematic analysis of qualitative information was completed systematically by coding data for the themes in practice and educational roles to summarize and describe clinical and educational activities [17].

3. Results

Of the 65 unique articles identified in PubMed and Embase, six studies met the inclusion criteria for analysis in this review [18–23]. The flowchart for inclusion and exclusion is provided in Figure 1. Of the six studies included, four studies occurred in the United States [18,19,21,23] and two studies occurred in Canada [20,22]. All of the included studies used similar survey methodology, including contacting FMRP program directors or their program administrators to identify the clinical pharmacists practicing within each FMRP. Each of the included studies used unique, researcher derived surveys with varying areas of focus for collecting data on pharmacists within FMRPs as noted in the data below. Surveys were not available for analysis.

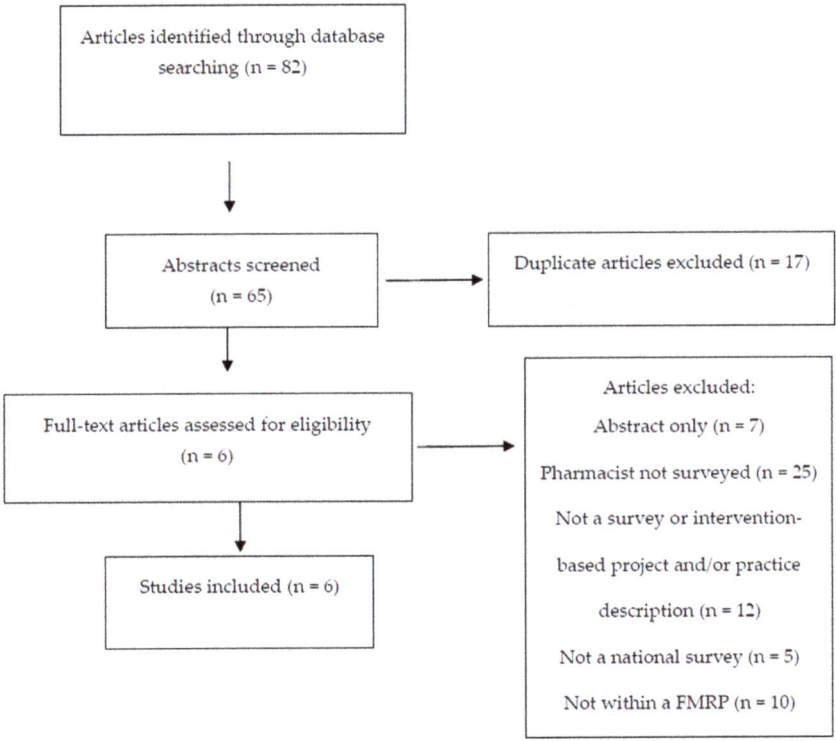

Figure 1. Flow diagram of the study.

3.1. Prevalence

The prevalence of clinical pharmacists in FMRPs has grown from 24% in 1990 to 53% in 2015 (95% CI 21.2–34.7; $p < 0.001$) in the United States [19,21,23] and from 14% in 1994 to 47% in 2009 (95% CI 17.6–45.1; $p < 0.001$) in Canada [20,22]. Table 1 describes the number of programs surveyed, program response rates, the number of programs with clinical pharmacists, and pharmacist survey response rates. The demographics of clinical pharmacists in FMRPs from 1983 to 2015 are described in Table 2. Overall, clinical pharmacists were young (<40 years old) with a PharmD degree, residency training, and had an appointment in a college/school of pharmacy or medicine.

Table 1. Clinical pharmacists in family medicine residency programs in North America from 1983 to 2015.

Survey Year (Country)	Total Number of Programs, n	Programs with Responses Obtained, n	Programs with Clinical Pharmacists, n	Programs with Pharmacists out of Programs with Responses, %	Pharmacist Survey Response Rate, %
2015 [23] (U.S.)	480	396	208	52.5 (208/396)	56.1 (142/253)
2009 [22] (Canada)	158	86	40	46.5 (40/86)	80.0 (32/40)
2000 [21] (U.S.)	579	555*	155	27.9 (155/555)	74.7 (130/174)
1994 [20] (Canada)	82	58	8	13.8 (8/58)	100.0 (9/9)
1990 [19] (U.S.)	381	325	79	24.3 (79/325)	NR
1983 [18] (U.S.)	386	NR	68	NR	72.1 (49/68)

Note: For the pharmacist survey response rate, the denominator represents the number of pharmacists identified from the programs with pharmacists. The numerator indicates the number of pharmacists responding to the survey. *Number was extrapolated from published data in each article, and was based on the calculation from response rate. U.S. = United States; NR = not reported.

Table 2. Demographics of clinical pharmacists in family medicine residency programs in North America from 1983 to 2015*.

Characteristic	1983 [18] (US), n = 49	1990 [19] (US), n = 80	1994 [20] (Canada), n = 9	2000 [21] (US), n = 130	2009 [22] (Canada), n = 32	2015 [23] (US), n = 142
Age, years	13 (27%) <30 29 (59%) 30–40 4 (8%) 41–50 3 (6%) 51–60 0 (0%) >60	34.6 (range 24–51)	"Most" were 30–40	36.5 ± 8.2 (range 25–59)	78% <45	38.5 ± 9.6 (range 26–67)
Gender Male Female	37 (76%) 12 (24%)	68% 32%	1 (11%) 8 (89%)	46% 54%	36% 65%	43 (30%) 99 (70%)
Degree PharmD	67%	85%	1 (11%)	89%	76%	138 (97%)
Residency	53%	68%	5 (56%)	69%	NR	104 (86%)
Academic appointment C/SOP C/SOM	28 (57%) 19 (39%)	61 (76%) 29 (36%)	NR NR	80% 52%	NR NR	105 (74%) 69 (49%)

*Reporting in the table varies based on how the data were reported in the studies. Underlined numbers were calculated based on the published data in each article. PharmD = doctor of pharmacy; C/SOP = college/school of pharmacy; C/SOM = college/school of medicine.

3.2. Clinical and Educational Scope

Within the Unites States, clinical pharmacists' time spent in direct patient care roles rose from 36% in 1990 to 53% in 2015, while time spent in teaching roles decreased from 43% in 2000 to 32% in 2015 [19,21,23]. The time clinical pharmacists in the United States reported spending on various areas within the FMRPs is shown in Table 3. The time Canadian clinical pharmacists spent was not described in the literature.

Regarding patient care activities, clinical pharmacists consistently provided patient education [18–20,22] and drug information [18–20,22,23]. Patient care services were reported in both inpatient [18,20,21,23] and outpatient settings [19–23]. The types of patient care activities reported include: inpatient rounding, direct patient care in outpatient practice, chart reviews, patient assistance programs, pharmacokinetic drug monitoring, nursing home visits and discharge counseling.

Clinical pharmacists within FMRPs have consistently provided clinical education through drug information [18–20,22,23] and indirect care activities, such as precepting, consults, and/or chart reviews [18–23]. Educational activities also often included formal teaching, such as didactic presentations and conferences [18,19,21–23] and also the noted facilitation of specific residency rotation for family medicine residents [19,21,23]. The learners consisted of family medicine residents [18–23] and pharmacy students [18–21,23]. Other interprofessional learners included medical students [19–21,23], nurses and nurse practitioners [18–21,23]. Pharmacy residents were first reported as learners in 2000 [21,23].

Table 3. Clinical pharmacist percentage of time spent within the United States family medicine residency programs.

	1990 [19]	2000 [21]	2015 [23]
Patient Care, %	36	37	53
Teaching, %	35	43	32
Research/Scholarship, %	12	12	8
Administration, %	NR	12	6

NR = not reported.

4. Discussion

Interprofessional education and training via clinical pharmacists as clinician educators within FMRPs is well established. This research sought to define the trends in the prevalence and clinical and educational scope over time within FMRPs in North America. Clinical pharmacists within FMRPs have grown significantly over the last 40 years in both the United States and Canada. The growth in integration of clinical pharmacists appears to have been through an expansion of their clinical and interprofessional teaching roles, with reductions in administrative and research time.

A swift growth in pharmacy residency training positions has supported this growth of clinical pharmacists within FMRPs. Post-graduate training for pharmacists has occurred since the 1930s with the official classification of residency training in the 1960s [24]. Pharmacy residency programs are delineated as post-graduate year 1 (PGY1) programs, which are general hospital practice-focused, or post-graduate year 2 (PGY2) programs, which are specialized in one area such as ambulatory care or critical care. Accredited PGY1 pharmacy residency programs have grown exponentially from roughly 1600 positions in 2007 to 3924 positions in 2020 [24,25]. Similarly, accredited ambulatory care PGY2 pharmacy residencies, the pharmacy specialty most congruent to family medicine, has grown from 62 positions in 2013 to 187 positions in 2020 [25]. In addition to clinical practice training and experience within residency training, many pharmacy residencies provide teaching experiences and faculty development [26,27]. The rapid growth of pharmacy residency programs for the training of clinical skills with an incorporation of teaching and faculty development has encouraged and supported the growth of competent clinician educators as pharmacists within FMRPs. Recently, the Accreditation Council for Graduate Medical Education (ACGME) expanded their medical residency faculty definition to include non-physician members, such as clinical pharmacists [28]. The scholarship, teaching, and education of clinical pharmacists within FMRPs now supports the overall FMRP faculty program requirements for accreditation.

Physician–pharmacist collaborative practices improve patient care outcomes and are cost effective [29]. Yet, barriers exist to the full integration of pharmacists into the care team, including perceptions of knowledge deficits, limited experience working with pharmacists, and communication challenges [30]. The integration of clinical pharmacists within FMRPs can invalidate many of these perceived barriers early in a physician's career, building the foundation for long-term, progressive incorporation of team-based care to improve patient outcomes, patient satisfaction, and provider satisfaction. Specifically, integrating clinical pharmacists may also help family medicine physicians and other members of the health care team meet the quadruple aims of improving population health, improving the patient's experience of care, reducing the per capita cost of health care, and improving the provider experience [31,32]. Pharmacists within FMRPs should share explicit information regarding their education, training, and benefits to their roles with physician residents and faculty to remove the perceived bias and implicit attitudes.

There are limitations to this systematic review of the literature. Each of the studies included in this review used different surveys for the collection of its data, making accurate comparisons challenging. Additionally, there are significant differences in healthcare and health-systems in the United States compared to Canada. While growth in team-based care is universal between the two countries, there are financial confounders in the U.S. related to the privatization of healthcare that limits the feasibility of the incorporation of clinical pharmacists within FMRPs.

The prevalence of clinical pharmacists within FMRPs in North America is growing. The education and training changes support clinical pharmacists as valuable clinicians for direct patient care and faculty members within FMRPs. The standardization of the integration of pharmacists within FMRPs supports training resident physicians to collaborate with pharmacists throughout their careers to improve patient outcomes in their practice.

5. Conclusions

The prevalence of clinical pharmacists in FMRPs is growing across North America. Clinical pharmacists are highly educated and trained to support these clinician educator positions.

Author Contributions: All authors participated in each aspect of the research and have read and agreed to the published version of the manuscript.

Funding: This research received no external funding.

Conflicts of Interest: The authors declare no conflict of interest.

References

1. American College of Clinical Pharmacy. Standards of Practice for Clinical Pharmacists. *Pharm. J. Hum. Pharmacol. Drug Ther.* **2014**, *34*, 794–797. [CrossRef] [PubMed]
2. Joint Comission of Pharmacy Practitioners. Pharmacists' Patient Care Process. Published Online 29 May 2014. Available online: https://jcpp.net/wp-content/uploads/2016/03/PatientCareProcess-with-supporting-organizations.pdf (accessed on 8 July 2020).
3. Branch, W.T.; Kroenke, K.; Levinson, W. The clinician-educator–present and future roles. *J. Gen. Intern. Med.* **1997**, *12* (Suppl. 2), S1–S4. [CrossRef] [PubMed]
4. Moore, T. Pharmacist faculty member in a family medicine residency program. *Am. J. Hosp. Pharm.* **1977**, *34*, 973–975. [CrossRef] [PubMed]
5. Love, D.; Hodge, N.; Foley, W. The clinical pharmacist in a family practice residency program. *J. Fam. Pract.* **1980**, *10*, 67–72. [PubMed]
6. Johnston, T.; Heffron, W. Clinical pharmacy in the family practice residency programs. *J. Fam. Pract.* **1981**, *13*, 91–94. [PubMed]
7. Haxby, D.; Weart, C.; Goodman, B. Family practice physicians' perceptions of the usefulness of drug therapy recommendations from clinical pharmacists. *Am. J. Hosp. Pharm.* **1988**, *45*, 824–827. [CrossRef]
8. Pottie, K.; Farrell, B.; Haydt, S.; Dolovich, L.; Sellors, C.; Kennie, N.; Hogg, W.; Martin, C.M. Integrating pharmacists into family practice teams: physicians' perspectives on collaborative care. *Can. Fam. Physician* **2008**, *54*, 1714–1717.

9. Jarrett, J.B.; Lounsbery, J.L.; D'Amico, F.; Dickerson, L.M.; Franko, J.; Nagle, J.; Seehusen, D.; Wilson, S.A. Clinical Pharmacists as Educators in Family Medicine Residency Programs: A CERA Study of Program Directors. *Fam. Med.* **2016**, *48*, 180–186.
10. Accreditation Standards and Key Elements for the Professional Program in Pharmacy Leading to the Doctor of Pharmacy Degree (Standards 2016). Published Online 2015. Available online: https://www.acpe-accredit.org/pdf/CS_PoliciesandProcedures.pdf (accessed on 2 May 2020).
11. Greiner, A.; Knebel, E. (Eds.) Institute of Medicine (US) Committee on The Health Professions Education Summit. Chapter 3, The Core Competencies Needed for Health Care Professionals. In *Professions Education: A Bridge. to Quality*; National Academies Press (US): Washington, DC, USA, 2003. Available online: https://www.ncbi.nlm.nih.gov/books/NBK221519/ (accessed on 7 April 2017).
12. Canadian Council for the Accreditation of Pharmacy Programs (CCAPP). Accreditation Standards for Canadian First Professional Degree in Pharmacy Programs. Published Online January 2018. Available online: http://ccapp-accredit.ca/wp-content/uploads/2016/01/Accreditation-Standards-for-Canadian-First-Professional-Degree-in-Pharmacy-Programs.pdf (accessed on 7 April 2017).
13. Canadian Hospital Pharmacy Residency Board. Accreditation Standards. Published Online January 2010. Available online: https://static1.squarespace.com/static/51b156fee4b0d15df77a6385/t/5329d58ae4b0e8b344d59962/1395250570379/CHPRB+Standards+FINAL+2010.pdf (accessed on 19 May 2020).
14. American Society of Health-System Pharmacists. ASHP Accreditation Standard for Postgraduate Year One (PGY1) Pharmacy Residency Programs. Published Online September 2016. Available online: https://www.ashp.org/-/media/assets/professional-development/residencies/docs/pgy1-accreditation-standard-2016.ashx?la=en&hash=82D0575273AD83E720B114D62B7926FD35792AFD (accessed on 7 April 2017).
15. Saseen, J.J.; Ripley, T.L.; Bondi, D.; Burke, J.M.; Cohen, L.J.; McBane, S.; McConnell, K.J.; Sackey, B.; Sanoski, C.; Simonyan, A.; et al. ACCP Clinical Pharmacist Competencies. *Pharm. J. Hum. Pharmacol. Drug Ther.* **2017**, *37*, 630–636. [CrossRef]
16. Moher, D.; Liberati, A.; Tetzlaff, J.; Altman, D.G. PRISMA Group. Preferred reporting items for systematic reviews and meta-analyses: The PRISMA statement. *PLoS Med.* **2009**, *6*, e1000097. [CrossRef]
17. Kiger, M.E.; Varpio, L. Thematic analysis of qualitative data: AMEE Guide No. 131. *Med. Teach.* **2020**, 1–9. [CrossRef] [PubMed]
18. Bendayan, R.; Robinson, J.D.; Stewart, R.B. Pharmaceutical services in family practice medical residency training programs. *Am. J. Hosp. Pharm.* **1983**, *40*, 274–277. [CrossRef] [PubMed]
19. Shaughnessy, A.F.; Hume, A.L. Clinical pharmacists in family practice residency programs. *J. Fam. Pract.* **1990**, *31*, 305–309. [PubMed]
20. Whelan, A.M.; Burge, F.; Munroe, K. Pharmacy services in family medicine residencies. Survey of clinics associated with Canadian residency programs. *Can. Fam. Physician* **1994**, *40*, 468–471.
21. Dickerson, L.M.; Denham, A.M.; Lynch, T. The state of clinical pharmacy practice in family practice residency programs. *Fam. Med.* **2002**, *34*, 653–657.
22. Jorgenson, D.; Muller, A.; Whelan, A.M.; Buxton, K. Pharmacists teaching in family medicine residency programs: National survey. *Can. Fam. Physician* **2011**, *57*, e341–e346.
23. Lounsbery, J.L.; Jarrett, J.B.; Dickerson, L.M.; Wilson, S.A. Integration of Clinical Pharmacists in Family Medicine Residency Programs. *Fam. Med.* **2017**, *49*, 430–436.
24. Johnson, T.J. Pharmacist work force in 2020: Implications of requiring residency training for practice. *Am. J. Health-Syst. Pharm.* **2008**, *65*, 166–170. [CrossRef]
25. National Matching Services Inc. ASHP Match Statistics (Updated 2020). 2020. Available online: https://natmatch.com/ashprmp/stats.html (accessed on 20 May 2020).
26. Strang, A.F.; Baia, P. An Investigation of Teaching and Learning Programs in Pharmacy Education. *Am. J. Pharm. Educ.* **2016**, *80*, 59. [CrossRef]
27. Havrda, D.E.; Engle, J.P.; Anderson, K.C.; Ray, S.M.; Haines, S.L.; Kane-Gill, S.L.; Ballard, S.L.; Crannage, A.J.; Rochester, C.D.; Parman, M.G.; et al. Guidelines for resident teaching experiences. *Pharmacotherapy* **2013**, *33*, e147–e161. [CrossRef]
28. Accreditation Council for Graduate Medical Education. ACGME Common Program Requirements (2017 Update). Available online: https://www.acgme.org/Portals/0/PFAssets/ProgramRequirements/CPRs_2017-07-01.pdf (accessed on 5 August 2018).

29. Hwang, A.Y.; Gums, T.H.; Gums, J.G. The benefits of physician-pharmacist collaboration. *J. Fam. Pract.* **2017**, *66*, E1–E8. [PubMed]
30. Patterson, B.J.; Solimeo, S.L.; Stewart, K.R.; Rosenthal, G.E.; Kaboli, P.J.; Lund, B.C. Perceptions of pharmacists' integration into patient-centered medical home teams. *Res. Soc. Adm. Pharm.* **2015**, *11*, 85–95. [CrossRef] [PubMed]
31. Bodenheimer, T.; Sinsky, C. From triple to quadruple aim: Care of the patient requires care of the provider. *Ann. Fam. Med.* **2014**, *12*, 573–576. [CrossRef] [PubMed]
32. Viswanathan, M.; Kahwati, L.C.; Golin, C.E.; Blalock, S.J.; Coker-Schwimmer, E.; Posey, R.; Lohr, K.N. Medication therapy management interventions in outpatient settings: A systematic review and meta-analysis. *JAMA Intern. Med.* **2015**, *175*, 76–87. [CrossRef] [PubMed]

© 2020 by the authors. Licensee MDPI, Basel, Switzerland. This article is an open access article distributed under the terms and conditions of the Creative Commons Attribution (CC BY) license (http://creativecommons.org/licenses/by/4.0/).

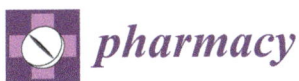

Review

The Evolving Role and Impact of Integrating Pharmacists into Primary Care Teams: Experience from Ontario, Canada

Manmeet Khaira [1,2], Annalise Mathers [1], Nichelle Benny Gerard [1] and Lisa Dolovich [1,2,3,*]

1. Leslie Dan Faculty of Pharmacy, University of Toronto, 144 College St, Toronto, ON M5S 3M2, Canada; manmeet.khaira@hotmail.com (M.K.); annalise.mathers@utoronto.ca (A.M.); nichelle.bennygerard@mail.utoronto.ca (N.B.G.)
2. School of Pharmacy, University of Waterloo, 10 Victoria St S, Kitchener, ON N2G 1C5, Canada
3. Department of Family Medicine, McMaster University, 1280 Main St W, Hamilton, ON L8S 4L8, Canada
* Correspondence: lisa.dolovich@utoronto.ca; Tel.: +1-416-978-3188

Received: 31 October 2020; Accepted: 5 December 2020; Published: 7 December 2020

Abstract: The movement to integrate pharmacists into primary care team-based settings is growing in countries such as Canada, the United States, the United Kingdom, and Australia. In the province of Ontario in Canada, almost 200 pharmacists have positions within interdisciplinary primary care team settings, including Family Health Teams and Community Health Centers. This article provides a narrative review of the evolving roles of pharmacists working in primary care teams, with a focus on evidence from Ontario, as well as drawing from other jurisdictions around the world. Pharmacists within primary care teams are uniquely positioned to facilitate the expansion of the pharmacist's scope of practice, through a collaborative care model that leverages, integrates, and transforms the medication expertise of pharmacists into a reliable asset and resource for physicians, as well as improves the health outcomes for patients and optimizes healthcare utilization.

Keywords: primary care team pharmacist; pharmacist-physician collaboration; comprehensive medication management; chronic care management; team-based primary care; interprofessional collaboration

1. Introduction

Although pharmacists are the most accessible and visited healthcare professionals in the world, the contributions that pharmacists make to interdisciplinary healthcare settings often remain overlooked [1–3]. It is known that poor communication and connectivity between healthcare professionals can fragment patient care, is a significant contributor to the development of drug-related problems (DRPs), and results in poorer health outcomes and experiences [4–6]. Moreover, since most prescribing of medications occurs in primary care, defined as a "whole-of-society approach to health and well-being" that addresses the broader determinants of health [7], pharmacists have an integral role in providing education and information about the appropriate and safe use of medications to patients, as well as to other healthcare professionals [8]. Healthcare professionals who work within a primary care team (PCT) have significantly improved communication and coordination, are optimally placed to detect and resolve DRPs, and can improve the availability and efficiency of healthcare [9,10].

In the past two decades, the movement to include pharmacists as essential members of PCTs has gained traction in a number of countries, including Canada [9,11,12], the United States [13–15], the United Kingdom [16,17], Australia [18], Malaysia [19–21], and Brazil [22]. Pharmacists integrated into interdisciplinary PCTs globally demonstrated their significant role in many direct patient care activities, including medication management, identifying adverse or incorrect medication usage, counselling on medications, and effectively optimizing a patient's understanding of their own medication regimens to enhance overall quality of life [9,23].

Canada has 10 provinces and 3 territories in which healthcare is primarily the responsibility of the province. In the province of Ontario, this is achieved with connection and coordination of the provincial healthcare system carried out by Ontario Health, an agency created by the Government of Ontario. Ontario recently transitioned to a regional health administrative structure with the introduction of Ontario Health Teams, which will eventually provide healthcare coverage for different areas of the province. Each Ontario Health Team is expected to provide integrated care across healthcare sectors, within a local community, including primary care. Primary care is provided through a mix of fee-for-service and organized-team-based care models. The most cohesive and comprehensive team-based care models are Family Health Teams (FHTs) and Community Health Centers. These provide care for approximately 20%, or 3 million people, in the province and are the main team-based setting, which include integrated primary care team pharmacists [24].

There are currently over 15,000 pharmacists working in Ontario (comprising approximately one-third of all pharmacists in Canada) [25] in pharmacy settings, including community, hospital, and interdisciplinary PCTs, such as FHTs and Community Health Centres [26]. Pharmacists are included as healthcare team members since the inception of the FHT model in Ontario in 2005. In FHTs, pharmacists provide on-site and in-office care to patients through specialized clinic services and comprehensive medication therapy management, and patient documentation by a pharmacist is included in the site electronic medical record [27]. Additionally within Canada, the province of British Columbia recently initiated a pilot program in 2018 to eventually integrate 50 pharmacists into PCTs, with the goal of revolutionizing pharmacy practice and patient care in that province [28]. Despite recent steps to embed pharmacists across Canada into PCTs, Canada lags behind other countries like the United Kingdom, where the National Health Service implemented a $100 million (in United States Dollars), five-year program to incorporate 1500 pharmacists into PCTs [17].

Given the continued expansion of pharmacy scope of practice in Ontario and across Canada, this article aims to provide a narrative review describing the evolution and evidence of the role of PCT pharmacists in Ontario, and then considers this evidence for the current impact of PCT pharmacists, in other jurisdictions around the world.

2. The Pharmacist's Role in Primary Care

The skills of pharmacists in primary care include the provision of direct patient care through management of medications, examination and screening, chronic disease management, drug information and education, collaboration and liaison, quality assurance, and research [29–31].

A study surveying pharmacists working in Ontario FHT sites about their involvement in various primary care activities found that the majority of time was spent on managing medications, conducting medication reviews, and communicating and educating other healthcare professionals (Table 1). As Ontario continues to see an expanded scope of practice, further research is required to determine how the activities of pharmacists in PCTs will also evolve.

Table 1. Selected major activities performed by pharmacists in Family Health Teams (FHTs) in Ontario [i].

Activity Category	Specific Activity Carried Out	Percent of Respondents N: % (N = 70)
Direct Patient Care	Managing medication-related issues	96
	General medication reviews	70
	Medication reconciliation	63
Education and drug information	Unstructured education to other healthcare practitioners	73
	Mentoring students	27
	Structured education to patients in a group setting	16
Systematic improvement programs	Creating new programs for patients	19
	Improvement in drug prescribing/use	17
Other activities	Research/quality improvement	9

[i] Adapted from [32].

In contrast to other pharmacy settings, pharmacists working in PCTs have additional roles that emerge when working with other healthcare professionals [33]. For example, pharmacists working in Ontario FHTs reported that their role was more strongly anchored in supporting healthcare professionals to manage medication use, locally implement national health priorities, arrange access to funding and health services, as well as design treatment pathways for patients [34]. The wider scope of a pharmacist's clinical duties in PCTs, which can include point of care anticoagulation monitoring in specialty PCT clinics, and direct collaboration with other healthcare professionals was shown to result in a longer acclimatization process for pharmacists in FHTs across Ontario, than for pharmacists in other practice settings [35]. However, research in Canada and the United Kingdom suggests that pharmacists working in primary care are well-positioned to build relationships with pharmacists working in community and hospital settings and ultimately collaborate to provide patient care that is coordinated across pharmacy settings. This might include monitoring of patients started on new medications, patients transitioning between healthcare environments, and improved accuracy and continuity of medication review assessments, and other healthcare information [36,37]. These intra-professional relationships and roles are critical to facilitate improved patient care. In the United Kingdom, a pilot project integrating nearly 1500 pharmacists into PCTs highlighted the additional roles of pharmacists responding to hospital discharges and prescribing, which, unlike in many other countries, pharmacists have the authority to do in the United Kingdom [38].

3. The Demonstrated Value of Pharmacists Integrated into PCTs

There is increasing evidence and support for the broader integration of pharmacists into PCTs. In Ontario, pharmacist integration into PCTs was shown to improve an array of health outcome quality measures, such as appropriate medication use, hypertension control, medication consultations, improved prescribing, reduced healthcare utilization and medication costs, and improvement in the management of chronic conditions [37]. The reductions in incorrect or unsafe use of medications quantify the direct benefits of the pharmacist's role into interdisciplinary PCTs and are further supported by research in Ontario, where pharmacists reported improved confidence in their role and the ability to support other healthcare professionals [10].

Identification of DRPs is one of the most significant contributions a PCT pharmacist can make. Research conducted across Ontario FHTs showed that medication reviews conducted by pharmacists are able to reduce medication discrepancies and rectify DRPs [6]. In this study, among a sample of 237 patients, 16 pharmacists found that patients were on an average of 9.2 prescription medications, and identified an average of 2.1 medication discrepancies and 3.6 DRPs per patient [6]. Pharmacists identified more than one medication discrepancy per patient and that almost every patient had a drug therapy problem. Similarly, in another Ontario study, when 7 pharmacists were integrated into seven PCTs and conducted medication reviews for 969 patients, PCT pharmacists were able to identify at least one DRP in 93.8% of patients, and also found an average of 4.4 DRPs per patient [37].

Another study of 1634 patients in an Ontario FHT identified DRPs in 88% of patients, with the most common DRPs categorized as additional drug therapy needed (33.7%), inappropriate dosage (16.1%), and adverse drug reactions (13.7%) [39]. When DRPs were identified by the PCT pharmacist, a positive clinical outcome was realized for approximately 80% of patients, upon 2-year follow-up [32]. These findings are comparable to findings across FHTs in Ontario that found the most common DRPs were additional drug therapy needed (22.6%), inappropriate dosage (14.1%), and receiving a drug with no indication (13.1%) [6]. In the province of Quebec, one study reported that pharmacists detected 300 DRPs (an average of 7.2 per patient) and that the most common DRP was 'drug use without indication' (27%); physicians accepted nearly 90% of the recommendations made by PCT pharmacists [9]. This is mirrored in Australia where PCT pharmacists have a higher rate of recommendations made and implemented, as a result of medication reviews, than those conducted by non-PCT pharmacists [40,41]. In another Australian study, the number of DRPs per patient fell to zero, after a 6-month follow-up with a PCT pharmacist, while patient adherence to medications simultaneously improved by approximately 20% [5].

These findings are further supported by a randomized control trial in Malaysia for patients with diabetes, hypertension, and hyperlipidemia, in which pharmacists were able to identify a medication issue in over 50% of patients [21]. Pharmacists were able to convey these issues to physicians, who implemented 87% of the pharmacist's recommendations [21]. Collectively, these findings demonstrate that pharmacists in PCTs are able to identify and address medication discrepancies and DRPs, to improve medication management, the provision of appropriate prescribing and simplifying patient's medication regimens.

The impact of pharmacist-led interventions in PCTs for elderly patients also improved medication adherence and reduced emergency room visits and hospitalizations due to DRPs [32], as well as improved prescribing appropriateness [42] in Ontario and globally. These improvements are particularly significant among polypharmacy patients [43]. Pharmacists in Ontario-based PCTs also showed improvements for chronic condition management among patients on medications for diabetes [44] and anticoagulation [35], which is also complemented by additional evidence from the province of Alberta, Canada, for improvements in blood pressure and cholesterol [45]. These studies demonstrate the pivotal and proactive role pharmacists play in optimizing patient care, when integrated into PCT settings around the world.

4. Collaboration with Physicians

Physicians attributed many benefits to having a pharmacist integrated into their practice, including having a colleague who is able to provide reliable drug information, optimize medication prescribing, improve clinical documentation, services, and recommendations, and enhance patient care [46]. In research conducted among physicians working in PCT sites across Ontario, physicians are supportive of receiving, and choosing to implement recommendations made by pharmacists working at the same PCT site [47]. In turn, PCT pharmacists reported receiving more consultations and referrals once the physician was offered initial feedback and suggestions regarding treatment plans for their patients [46–48]. At Women's College Hospital in Toronto, collaboration between a clinical pharmacist, a pharmacy resident, and physicians, allowed the interdisciplinary team to successfully meet their deprescribing goal, aligned with the World Health Organization's call for action to decrease avoidable medication-related harm [49]. This collaboration between physicians and pharmacists also led to improved relationships and communication between healthcare professionals that facilitate patient care planning, documentation, and implementation [33].

In the state of California in the United States, 69 physicians participated in a cross-sectional survey on their experience working with clinical pharmacists in PCTs; 90% of physicians noted improved medication management of their patients and 93% of respondents recognized the pharmacist's recommendations as clinically meaningful [15]. Similarly, in a survey of fifty-six physicians in the state of North Carolina, 87.5% felt that identifying enhanced clinical outcomes was the top benefit of embedding a clinical pharmacist into their practice [50]. In addition to optimizing outcomes for patients, a systematic review found that pharmacists in PCTs reduced physician workload substantially [51]. Primary care physicians further described that the inclusion of a clinical pharmacist can improve the perceived quality of their patients' healthcare, the quality of the medication decisions made, and the management of medications [29]. Patients who met with both a physician and pharmacist when transitioning between points of care, for example, from hospital to home, reported a reduced hospital readmission rate as well as benefitted from discontinuing an unnecessary medication, receiving new medications, and having non-adherence addressed [29].

In jurisdictions such as Malaysia where pharmacist integration is emerging, it is important to leverage evidence from countries where integration of pharmacists was successful, in order to strengthen physician awareness of and support for the significant roles and contributions of pharmacists in PCTs [19,20].

5. Perspectives from Patients

The benefit of pharmacists in primary healthcare was also studied among patients. At the Centre for Family Medicine Family Health Team in Ontario, patients and caregivers communicated the benefits of having a comprehensive medication review in an interdisciplinary setting. This includes a decrease in inappropriate medication use, optimization of hypertension and diabetes medication regimens, as well as minimization of antipsychotic use for the behavioral and psychiatric symptoms of dementia [33]. In the United States, pharmacist-managed clinics act as an opportunity for patients to receive detailed medication information, focused on their specific needs and desires [52]. Patients expressed a sense of companionship with the pharmacist, which improved the patient's desire to reach their healthcare goals [52]. In Malaysia, qualitative research on patient perspectives on pharmacist integration demonstrates that patients believe pharmacists play a substantial role in informing patients of the safe and appropriate use of medications [19]. Additionally, when PCT pharmacists provide medication education and information, many patients feel that the medication-related education, disease-related education, and delivery of education they receive is excellent [53]. Research around the world supports that patients prefer to have their care coordinated between a physician and pharmacist and recognize that this collaboration is integral to optimizing their care [5].

6. Evolving Pharmacy Education and Practice

The role, impact, and value that pharmacists contribute to primary care is significant. In order to support the continued integration of pharmacists into PCTs, improvements in educational and training opportunities for young pharmacists is required globally [10,22]. The "ADapting pharmacists' skills and Approaches to maximize Patient's drug Therapy effectiveness" (ADAPT) program was developed based on experience with training and mentoring pharmacists, to integrate into PCTs in Ontario and that hosted by the Canadian Pharmacists Association [54–57]. The ADAPT program aimed to provide a standard approach to medication assessment, team collaboration, patient assessment, evidence-based decision making, and documentation, facilitated through an e-learning program [57–59]. This program provided evidence supporting continuing education via online learning, with pharmacists reporting high satisfaction and confidence in skills that they could directly apply in their professional careers [57,58]. The ADAPT educational program was adapted for use by clinical pharmacists and professors at the Virginia Commonwealth University School of Pharmacy in the state of Virginia, United States. Its use resulted in improvements in providing care, interviewing, documenting, and collaboration for pharmacists working within primary care in Canada and the United States [60].

Research from the existing Primary Care Pharmacy Specialty Network (PC-PSN) in Canada also demonstrated that listservs can act as key channels for PCT pharmacists to connect to share information, identify solutions for complex patients and care, and provide mentorship opportunities [61]. Further research demonstrates that pharmacists identified key competencies for working in primary care, which include a focus on communication, collaboration, and professionalism, and consider how these relate to pharmacists and other healthcare professionals in understanding the evolving roles of PCT pharmacists in order to establish performance indicators to support professional education [62]. As found in Brazil, training opportunities within interprofessional teams also improves the understanding that healthcare professionals have about the roles and competencies of pharmacists on their PCT, and in the long-term can help to demonstrate the impact and importance of their work [22]. To complement this work, opportunities for pharmacists to gain direct experience through training and educational placements in PCT environments, and to continue to build a community that fosters sharing of interprofessional clinical knowledge and skills, will better equip pharmacists for future practice in PCT environments.

To strengthen the successful integration of pharmacists into PCT practice settings, is it critical to ensure there are opportunities and support available for the increased visibility of pharmacists as PCT ambassadors. For example, in Ontario, at times a pharmacist represents allied healthcare professionals on the Association of Family Health Teams Ontario (AFHTO) Board of Directors, which improves the visibility and credibility for the role of pharmacists in PCTs [26]. Furthermore, the Pharmacy Specialty Network (PSN) developed by the Canadian Society of Hospital Pharmacists and the Canadian Pharmacists Association, enables pharmacists to share practice-based resources; develop, support, and maintain networking opportunities for pharmacists; advocate for the role of pharmacists in PCTs; and provide education and training to its members, including mentorship opportunities for pharmacists new to PCT settings [63]. The development of Pharmacist Program Toolkits by the IMPACT project (Integrating Family Medicine and Pharmacy to Advance Primary Care Therapeutics; www.impactteam.info) provides guidance and strategies for PCTs to successfully integrate pharmacists alongside other healthcare professionals. To provide additional resources for PCT pharmacists, the Ontario Pharmacists Association developed a toolkit [64] that pharmacists can leverage to practice to their full scope.

7. Improved Outcomes for Patients and Optimization of Health Systems

A systematic review found that emergency room visits decreased and savings in medication and health system costs were realized when pharmacists are integrated into PCTs, even with increased primary care usage [51]. Improvements in health outcomes at the individual and population level was also demonstrated when pharmacists work as a member of an inter-professional team, as well as decreased fragmentation within the healthcare system [51]. Although there are no published economics analyses based on the Ontario data, one study estimates that PCT pharmacists can offset costs to the healthcare system by $1079 per patient and can generate revenues for the PCT that are 38% in excess of the cost of the pharmacist's time [29]. To realize these opportunities more fully in primary care in Ontario and around the world, further research is required to evaluate health system impacts and outcomes, over the long-term, upon embedding pharmacists into PCTs.

8. Conclusions

Pharmacists in Ontario are now formally funded by the public healthcare system to be members of the interdisciplinary healthcare team. There is a growing evidence base that describes the role and impact of Ontario-based PCT pharmacists, which is consistent with evidence emerging worldwide. Pharmacists within PCTs are uniquely positioned to facilitate the expansion of the pharmacist's scope of practice through a collaborative care model that leverages, integrates, and transforms the medication expertise of pharmacists into a reliable asset and resource for physicians. Further research in Ontario is needed to quantify the effectiveness of PCT pharmacists on health outcomes, and the resulting impact on healthcare service use and costs.

Author Contributions: Conceptualization, L.D. and M.K.; methodology, L.D. and M.K.; formal analysis, L.D., M.K., A.M., and N.B.G.; investigation, L.D., M.K., A.M., and N.B.G.; data curation, M.K., A.M., and N.B.G.; writing—Original draft preparation, M.K.; writing—Review and editing, L.D., M.K., A.M., and N.B.G.; supervision, L.D.; project administration, L.D.; funding acquisition, L.D. All authors have read and agreed to the published version of the manuscript.

Funding: This research results from an Applied Health Research Question submitted by The Association of Family Health Teams (AFHTO) to the Ontario Pharmacy Evidence Network (OPEN). OPEN was funded by a grant from the Government of Ontario (grant #6674). The views expressed in this manuscript are those of the authors and do not necessarily reflect those of the funder.

Acknowledgments: The authors would like to acknowledge the contributions of Divjyot Kochar who helped with aspects of writing review and editing.

Conflicts of Interest: The authors declare no conflict of interest.

References

1. Manolakis, P.G.; Skelton, J.B. Pharmacists' contributions to primary care in the United States collaborating to address unmet patient care needs: The emerging role for pharmacists to address the shortage of primary care providers. *Am. J. Of Pharm. Educ.* **2010**, *74*. [CrossRef] [PubMed]
2. YOUR RPS. The changing role of the pharmacist in the 21st century. *Pharm. J.* **2018**, *300*. Available online: https://www.pharmaceutical-journal.com/your-rps/the-changing-role-of-the-pharmacist-in-the-21st-century/20204131.article?firstPass=false (accessed on 30 November 2020). [CrossRef]
3. Bauman, J.L. Hero clinical pharmacists and the COVID-19 pandemic: Overworked and overlooked. *J. Am. Coll. Clin. Pharm.* **2020**. [CrossRef] [PubMed]
4. Tan, E.; Stewart, K.; Elliott, R.A.; George, J. An exploration of the role of pharmacists within general practice clinics: The protocol for the pharmacists in practice study (PIPS). *BMC Health Serv. Res.* **2012**, *12*, 1–6. [CrossRef]
5. Tan, E.C.; Stewart, K.; Elliott, R.A.; George, J. Pharmacist consultations in general practice clinics: The Pharmacists in Practice Study (PIPS). *Res. Soc. Adm. Pharm.* **2014**, *10*, 623–632. [CrossRef]
6. Benny Gerard, N.; Mathers, A.; Laeer, C.; Lui, E.; Kontio, T.; Patel, P.; Dolovich, L. A Descriptive Quantitative Analysis on the Extent of Polypharmacy in Recipients of Ontario Primary Care Team Pharmacist-Led Medication Reviews. *Pharmacy* **2020**, *8*, 110. [CrossRef]
7. World Health Organization. Primary Health Care. Available online: https://www.google.com/url?q=https://www.who.int/health-topics/primary-health-care%23tab%3Dtab_1&sa=D&ust=1606175083856000&usg=AOvVaw37ze4hWcsshb-K2NgY0WCp (accessed on 24 November 2020).
8. Canadian Patient Safety Institute. Medication Safety. 2020. Available online: https://www.patientsafetyinstitute.ca/en/Topic/Pages/Medication-Safety.aspx (accessed on 23 January 2020).
9. Abdin, M.S.; Grenier-Gosselin, L.; Guénette, L. Impact of pharmacists' interventions on the pharmacotherapy of patients with complex needs monitored in multidisciplinary primary care teams. *Int. J. Pharm. Pract.* **2020**, *28*, 75–83. [CrossRef]
10. Butterworth, J.; Sansom, A.; Sims, L.; Healey, M.; Kingsland, E.; Campbell, J. Pharmacists' perceptions of their emerging general practice roles in UK primary care: A qualitative interview study. *Br. J. Gen. Pract.* **2017**, *67*, e650–e658. [CrossRef]
11. Jorgenson, D.; Dalton, D.; Farrell, B.; Tsuyuki, R.T.; Dolovich, L. Guidelines for pharmacists integrating into primary care teams. *Can. Pharm. J. Rev. Pharm. Can.* **2013**, *146*, 342–352. [CrossRef]
12. Raiche, T.; Pammett, R.; Dattani, S.; Dolovich, L.; Hamilton, K.; Kennie-Kaulbach, N.; McCarthy, L.; Jorgenson, D. Community pharmacists' evolving role in Canadian primary health care: A vision of harmonization in a patchwork system. *Pharm. Pract.* **2020**, *18*, 2171. [CrossRef]
13. Jacobi, J. Clinical pharmacists: Practitioners who are essential members of your clinical care team. *Rev. Méd. Clín. Condes* **2016**, *27*, 571–577. [CrossRef]
14. Chisholm-Burns, M.A.; Lee, J.K.; Spivey, C.A.; Slack, M.; Herrier, R.N.; Hall-Lipsy, E.; Zivin, J.G.; Abraham, I.; Palmer, J. US pharmacists' effect as team members on patient care: Systematic review and meta-analyses. *Med. Care* **2010**, 923–933. [CrossRef] [PubMed]
15. Moreno, G.; Lonowski, S.; Fu, J.; Chon, J.S.; Whitemire, N.; Vasquez, C.; Skootsky, S.A.; Bell, D.S.; Maranon, R.; Mangione, C.M. Physician experiences with clinical pharmacists in primary care teams. *J. Am. Pharm. Assoc. JAPhA* **2017**, *57*, 686–691. [CrossRef]
16. Silcock, J.; Raynor, D.K.; Petty, D. The organisation and development of primary care pharmacy in the United Kingdom. *Health Policy* **2004**, *67*, 207–214. [CrossRef]
17. NHS England. General Practice Forward View. Available online: https://www.england.nhs.uk/wp-content/uploads/2016/04/gpfv.pdf (accessed on 15 August 2018).
18. Moles, R.J.; Stehlik, P. Pharmacy practice in Australia. *Can. J. Hosp. Pharm.* **2015**, *68*, 418. [CrossRef] [PubMed]
19. San Saw, P.; Nissen, L.M.; Freeman, C.; Wong, P.S.; Mak, V. Health care consumers' perspectives on pharmacist integration into private general practitioner clinics in Malaysia: A qualitative study. *Patient Prefer. Adherence* **2015**, *9*, 467. [CrossRef]
20. Saw, P.S.; Nissen, L.; Freeman, C.; Wong, P.S.; Mak, V. A qualitative study on pharmacists' perception on integrating pharmacists into private general practitioner's clinics in Malaysia. *Pharm. Pract.* **2017**, *15*.

21. Chua, S.S.; Kok, L.C.; Yusof, F.A.M.; Tang, G.H.; Lee, S.W.H.; Efendie, B.; Paraidathathu, T. Pharmaceutical care issues identified by pharmacists in patients with diabetes, hypertension or hyperlipidaemia in primary care settings. *Bmc Health Serv. Res.* **2012**, *12*, 388. [CrossRef]
22. Barberato, L.C.; Scherer, M.D.D.A.; Lacourt, R.M.C. The pharmacist in the Brazilian Primary Health Care: Insertion under construction. *Ciênc. Saúde Colet.* **2019**, *24*, 3717–3726. [CrossRef]
23. Wells, W.D. Pharmacists are key members of primary healthcare teams. *BMJ Br. Med. J.* **1997**, *314*, 1486. [CrossRef]
24. Ministry of Health and Long-Term Care. Family Health Teams. 2016. Available online: http://www.health.gov.on.ca/en/pro/programs/fht/ (accessed on 29 October 2020).
25. National Association of Pharmacy Regulatory Authorities (NAPRA). National Statistics. Available online: https://napra.ca/national-statistics (accessed on 21 October 2020).
26. AFHTO, Association of Family Health Teams of Ontario. Five Things You Need to Know About Family Health Team Pharmacists. Available online: https://www.afhto.ca/news-events/news/five-things-you-need-know-about-family-health-team-pharmacists (accessed on 23 January 2020).
27. Dolovich, L. Ontario pharmacists practicing in family health teams and the patient-centered medical home. *Ann. Pharmacother.* **2012**, *46*, 33S–39S. [CrossRef] [PubMed]
28. Gobis, B.; Zed, P.J. The journey begins: BC roadmap for pharmacist integration into team-based primary care. *Can. Pharm. J.* **2020**, *153*, 141–143. [CrossRef]
29. Scott, M.A.; Heck, J.E.; Wilson, C.G. The integral role of the clinical pharmacist practitioner in primary care. *North Carol. Med. J.* **2017**, *78*, 181–185. [CrossRef] [PubMed]
30. Benson, H.; Lucas, C.; Benrimoj, S.I.; Williams, K.A. The development of a role description and competency map for pharmacists in an interprofessional care setting. *Int. J. Clin. Pharm.* **2019**, *41*, 391–407. [CrossRef] [PubMed]
31. Giannitrapani, K.F.; Glassman, P.A.; Vang, D.; McKelvey, J.C.; Day, R.T.; Dobscha, S.K.; Lorenz, K.A. Expanding the role of clinical pharmacists on interdisciplinary primary care teams for chronic pain and opioid management. *BMC Fam. Pract.* **2018**, *19*, 107. [CrossRef] [PubMed]
32. Gillespie, U.; Dolovich, L.; Dahrouge, S. Activities performed by pharmacists integrated in family health teams: Results from a web-based survey. *Can. Pharm. J.* **2017**, *150*, 407–416. [CrossRef] [PubMed]
33. The College of Family Physicians of Canada and the Canadian Pharmacists Association. Innovation in Primary Care: Integration of Pharmacists into Interprofessional Teams. Available online: https://www.cfpc.ca/uploadedFiles/Health_Policy/IPC-2019-Pharmacist-Integration.pdf (accessed on 20 April 2019).
34. Royal Pharmaceutical Society. Primary Care Pharmacy. Available online: https://www.rpharms.com/resources/careers-information/career-options-in-pharmacy/primary-care-pharmacy (accessed on 23 January 2020).
35. Rossiter, J.; Soor, G.; Telner, D.; Aliarzadeh, B.; Lake, J. A pharmacist-led point-of-care INR clinic: Optimizing care in a family health team setting. *Int. J. Fam. Med.* **2013**, *2013*, 701. [CrossRef]
36. Cymru, W.; Royal Pharmaceutical Society; NHS Wales. Models of Care for Pharmacy within Primary Care Clusters. Available online: http://www.gpun.cymru.nhs.uk/sitesplus/documents/1000/Models%20of%20Care%20for%20Pharmacy%20within%20Primary%20Care%20Clusters_Final1.pdf (accessed on 23 January 2020).
37. Dolovich, L.; Pottie, K.; Kaczorowski, J.; Farrell, B.; Austin, Z.; Rodriguez, C.; Gaebel, K.; Sellors, C. Integrating family medicine and pharmacy to advance primary care therapeutics. *Clin. Pharmacol. Ther.* **2008**, *83*, 913–917. [CrossRef]
38. Komwong, D.; Greenfield, G.; Zaman, H.; Majeed, A.; Hayhoe, B. Clinical pharmacists in primary care: A safe solution to the workforce crisis? *J. R. Soc. Med.* **2018**, *111*, 120–124. [CrossRef]
39. Lui, E.; Ha, R.; Truong, C. Applying the pharmaceutical care model to assess pharmacist services in a primary care setting. *Can. Pharm. J.* **2017**, *150*, 90–93. [CrossRef]
40. Freeman, C.R.; Cottrell, W.N.; Kyle, G.; Williams, I.D.; Nissen, L. An evaluation of medication review reports across different settings. *Int. J. Clin. Pharm.* **2013**, *35*, 5–13. [CrossRef] [PubMed]
41. Sorensen, L.; Stokes, J.A.; Purdie, D.M.; Woodward, M.; Elliott, R.; Roberts, M.S. Medication reviews in the community: Results of a randomized, controlled effectiveness trial. *Br. J. Clin. Pharmacol.* **2004**, *58*, 648–664. [CrossRef] [PubMed]

42. Riordan, D.O.; Walsh, K.A.; Galvin, R.; Sinnott, C.; Kearney, P.M.; Byrne, S. The effect of pharmacist-led interventions in optimising prescribing in older adults in primary care: A systematic review. *Sage Open Med.* **2016**, *4*, 2050312116652568. [CrossRef] [PubMed]
43. Hazen, A.C.; De Bont, A.A.; Boelman, L.; Zwart, D.L.; De Gier, J.J.; De Wit, N.J.; Bouvy, M.L. The degree of integration of non-dispensing pharmacists in primary care practice and the impact on health outcomes: A systematic review. *Res. Soc. Adm. Pharm.* **2018**, *14*, 228–240. [CrossRef]
44. Gagnon, A.; Jin, M.; Malak, M.; Bednarowski, K.; Feng, L.; Francis-Pringle, S.; Lu, S.; Mallin, A.; Skokovic-Sunij, D.; Vedelago, A. Pharmacists Managing People with Diabetes in Primary Care: 10 Years of Experience at the Hamilton Family Health Team. *Can. J. Diabetes* **2017**, *41*, 576. [CrossRef]
45. Simpson, S.H.; Majumdar, S.R.; Tsuyuki, R.T.; Lewanczuk, R.Z.; Spooner, R.; Johnson, J.A. Effect of adding pharmacists to primary care teams on blood pressure control in patients with type 2 diabetes: A randomized controlled trial. *Diabetes Care* **2011**, *34*, 20–26. [CrossRef]
46. Kennie, N.; Farrell, B.; Dolovich, L. Demonstrating Value, Documenting Care: Lessons Learned about Writing Comprehensive Patient Medication Assessments in the IMPACT Project: Part I: Getting Started with Documenting Medication Assessments. *Can. Pharm. J.* **2008**, *141*, 114–119. [CrossRef]
47. Farrell., B.; Dolovich, L.; Austin, Z.; Sellors, C. Implementing a mentorship program for pharmacists integrating into family practice: Practical experience from the IMPACT project team. *Can. Pharm. J.* **2010**, *143*, 28–36. [CrossRef]
48. Truong, C.; Ha, R.; Lui, E. Hybrid model of pharmacist services in a large multisite family health team. *Can. Pharm. J.* **2020**, *153*, 270–273. [CrossRef]
49. Raiche, T.; Visentin, J.D.; Fernandes, L. Quality Improvement: A strategy to accelerate pharmacist integration into team-based primary practice. *Can. Pharm. J.* **2020**, *153*, 274–279. [CrossRef]
50. Williams, C.R.; Woodall, T.; Wilson, C.G.; Griffin, R.; Galvin, S.L.; LaVallee, L.A.; Roberts, C.; Ives, T.J. Physician perceptions of integrating advanced practice pharmacists into practice. *J. Am. Pharm. Assoc. JAPhA* **2018**, *58*, 73–78. [CrossRef]
51. Hayhoe, B.; Cespedes, J.A.; Foley, K.; Majeed, A.; Ruzangi, J.; Greenfield, G. Impact of integrating pharmacists into primary care teams on health systems indicators: A systematic review. *Br. J. Gen. Pract.* **2019**, *69*, e665–e674. [CrossRef] [PubMed]
52. Gonzalvo, J.D.; Papineau, E.C.; Ramsey, D.C.; Vincent, A.H.; Walton, A.M.; Weber, Z.A.; Wilhoite, J.E. Patient Perceptions of Pharmacist-Managed Clinics: A Qualitative Analysis. *J. Pharm. Technol.* **2012**, *28*, 10–15. [CrossRef]
53. Knight, D.E.; Caudill, J.A.L. Implementation of a patient perception survey in a pharmacist-managed primary care clinic and analysis with a unique HFMEA method. *J. Am. Pharm. Assoc.* **2010**, *50*, 78–85a. [CrossRef] [PubMed]
54. Farrell, B.; Pottie, K.; Haydt, S.; Kennie, N.; Sellors, C.; Dolovich>, L. Integrating into family practice: The experiences of pharmacists in Ontario, Canada. *Int. J. Pharm. Pract.* **2008**, *16*, 309–315. [CrossRef]
55. Lau, E.; Dolovich, L.; Austin, Z. Comparison of self, physician, and simulated patient ratings of pharmacist performance in a family practice simulator. *J. Interprof. Care* **2007**, *21*, 129–140. [CrossRef] [PubMed]
56. Austin, Z.; Dolovich, L.; Lau, E.; Tabak, D.; Sellors, C.; Marini, A.; Kennie, N. Teaching and Assessing Primary Care Skills: The Family Practice Simulator Model. *Am. J. Pharm. Educ.* **2005**, *69*, 500–507. [CrossRef]
57. Farrell, B.; Ward, N.; Jennings, B.; Jones, C.; Jorgenson, D.; Gubbels-Smith, A.; Dolovich, L.; Kennie, N. Participation in online continuing education. *Int. J. Pharm. Pract.* **2016**, *24*, 60–71. [CrossRef]
58. Farrell, B.; Jennings, B.; Ward, N.; Marks, P.Z.; Kennie, N.; Dolovich, L.; Jordenson, D.; Jones, C.; Gubbels, A. Evaluation of a pilot e-learning primary health care skills training program for pharmacists. *Curr. Pharm. Teach. Learn.* **2013**, *5*, 580–592. [CrossRef]
59. Farrell, B.; Dolovich, L.; Emberley, P.; Gagné, M.A.; Jennings, B.; Jorgenson, D.; Kennie, N.; Marks, P.Z.; Pzpoushek, C.; Waite, N.; et al. Designing a novel continuing education program for pharmacists: Lessons learned. *Can. Pharm. J.* **2012**, *145*, e7–e16. [CrossRef]
60. Moczygemba, L.R.; Pierce, A.L.; Dang, A.; Emberley, P.; Czar, M.J.; Matzke, G.R. The ADAPT online education program: A tool for practicing pharmacists delivering patient-centered care. *J. Am. Pharm. Assoc.* **2017**, *57*, 601–607. [CrossRef] [PubMed]

61. Trinacty, M.; Farrell, B.; Schindel, T.J.; Sunstrum, L.; Dolovich, L.; Kennie, N.; Russell, G.; Waite, N. Learning and networking: Utilization of a primary care listserv by pharmacists. *Can. J. Hosp. Pharm.* **2014**, *67*, 343–352. [CrossRef] [PubMed]
62. Kennie-Kaulbach, N.; Farrell, B.; Ward, N.; Johnston, S.; Gubbels, A.; Eguale, T.; Dolovich, L.; Jorgenson, D.; Waite, N.; Winslade, N. Pharmacist provision of primary health care: A modified Delphi validation of pharmacists' competencies. *BMC Fam. Pract.* **2012**, *13*, 27. [CrossRef] [PubMed]
63. CSHP/CPhA Primary Care Pharmacists Pharmacy Specialty Network (PSN) Terms of Reference. Available online: http://www.impactteam.info/documents/PSNTermsofReferenceoctober2007_000.pdf (accessed on 23 January 2020).
64. Ontario Pharmacists Association. OPA Family Health Team Resource Kit. Available online: http://www.impactteam.info/documents/fht_toolkit.pdf (accessed on 21 October 2020).

Publisher's Note: MDPI stays neutral with regard to jurisdictional claims in published maps and institutional affiliations.

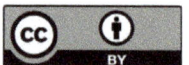

© 2020 by the authors. Licensee MDPI, Basel, Switzerland. This article is an open access article distributed under the terms and conditions of the Creative Commons Attribution (CC BY) license (http://creativecommons.org/licenses/by/4.0/).

MDPI
St. Alban-Anlage 66
4052 Basel
Switzerland
Tel. +41 61 683 77 34
Fax +41 61 302 89 18
www.mdpi.com

Pharmacy Editorial Office
E-mail: pharmacy@mdpi.com
www.mdpi.com/journal/pharmacy

www.ingramcontent.com/pod-product-compliance
Lightning Source LLC
LaVergne TN
LVHW070542100526
838202LV00012B/354